# Your Teaching Style

## A practical guide to understanding, developing and improving

Kay Mohanna FRCGP, PGDipMedEd, MA
*Principal Lecturer in Medical Education, Staffordshire University*
*Associate Dean, West Midlands Workforce Deanery*

Ruth Chambers FRCGP, DM
*Director of Postgraduate GP Education, West Midlands Workforce Deanery*

and

David Wall MMEd, PhD, FRCP, FRCGP
*Deputy Postgraduate Dean, West Midlands Workforce Deanery*
*Honorary Professor of Medical Education, Staffordshire University*

Radcliffe Publishing
Oxford • New York

**Radcliffe Publishing Ltd**
18 Marcham Road
Abingdon
Oxon OX14 1AA
United Kingdom

**www.radcliffe-oxford.com**
Electronic catalogue and worldwide online ordering facility.

British Library Cataloguing in Publication Data

A catalogue record for this book is available from the British Library.

ISBN-13: 978 1 85775 858 0

Typeset by Phoenix Photosetting, Chatham, Kent
Printed and bound by TJ International Ltd, Padstow, Cornwall

# Your Teaching Style

A practical guide to understanding, developing and improving

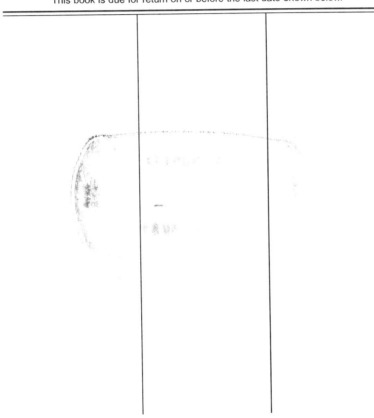

# Contents

# Preface

We have said before that the credit for many of the insights we use when writing and teaching about learning and teaching should in fact be given to our own teachers in our study of medical education.

We have also said that:

> it would be impossible to name all the influences [on us as teachers] even if we could tease out who had taught us what. If you recognise your words in our work, you were a good teacher. Thank you.[1]

This applies even more so to developing our thinking about teaching styles. Each of us remembers inspirational teachers who have drawn us into the study of medical education. In addition we also recall examples of such appalling lack of match between our preferred learning style and the teaching style of our teachers that we determined to do better ourselves. Only our students know if we succeed more often than we fail in that aim.

There is a changing culture towards development of a 'learning environment' in the health service. There are many new learning requirements in the modern National Health Service (NHS) and much that has to be learned will be about attitudes and beliefs in addition to knowledge and skills. Traditional learning activities (e.g. in the lecture theatre) can be less helpful for such domains of learning. We are seeing an increase in the amount of learning in teams and, as novices to this way of learning, teams may need some help to get going with development of team leaders as facilitators of learning. The emphasis on access, both to care and to learning opportunities, within the NHS also means that teachers will need to be able to motivate and teach a new set of mature health professionals who may require different types of support from their teachers.

This book is based on our original research looking at effective teaching. We have devised a self assessment questionnaire to determine your preferred teaching style and aim to provide tips and advice that can be integrated into your everyday teaching and learning practice. We hope it will enable you to plan to improve your teaching skills and enhance your effectiveness as a teacher.

**Kay Mohanna**
*October 2007*

# Reference

1    Mohanna K, Wall D, Chambers R. *Teaching Made Easy: a manual for health professionals*. 2nd ed. Oxford: Radcliffe Medical Press; 2004.

# About the authors

**Kay Mohanna** is a principal in general practice and a GP trainer for undergraduates and postgraduate doctors in training. She is also principal lecturer in medical education at Staffordshire University where she has developed and run the MSc in medical education for the past eight years. She is an external examiner at Warwick University and is an associate dean at the West Midlands Workforce Deanery for assessment in GP specialty training. Currently Vice Chair of the Royal College of General Practitioners Midland Faculty, she was previously the education convenor and was responsible for the West Midlands GP Appraisal Support Programme. Her particular interest in teaching is in faculty development and she has a research interest in evaluation of teaching. She has worked with and listened to lots of learners in a variety of settings and this work on teaching styles partly arose from those discussions.

**Ruth Chambers** has been a GP for 25 years and still practises part-time. She is the director of postgraduate general practice education at NHS West Midlands Strategic Health Authority, Professor of Health Development at Staffordshire University and national education lead for the NHS Alliance. She has made lots of mistakes in teaching and training repeated less often as the years have gone by. Ruth has given and organised many lectures, workshops and seminars for small groups and vast numbers of people. She has run several series of learner sets, as well as written and organised a distance learning course. Her Doctorate included research about the ways that health professionals apply new knowledge in practice. Ruth and others have written a series of books for doctors and nurses to help them to prepare and collect evidence of their competence and performance in their everyday work, whatever their specialty.

**David Wall** is deputy regional postgraduate dean in the West Midlands Workforce Deanery and honorary professor of medical education at Staffordshire University. He has been deputy postgraduate dean since1996, having previously been the regional adviser for general practice. He has been a general practitioner in Four Oaks in Sutton Coldfield for 30 years. He is also external examiner for the University of Dundee, and has just finished five years as external examiner with the University of Plymouth and Peninsula Medical School. He obtained a diploma in medical education from the University of Dundee in 1996 and a Masters Degree in medical education from the University of Dundee in 1998. He has obtained a PhD in Education from the University of Birmingham, on the effects of educational qualifications on the work of medical educators. His research interests include curriculum studies, teaching the teachers, assessment of behaviours and anything else in medical education that seems an interesting research question to try to answer.

# Chapter 1

# The importance of variation in teaching styles

*Kay Mohanna*

Recommendations to novice healthcare teachers about effective teaching of the 'how to do it' variety, tend to be based on the obvious ('prepare well'), personal opinion ('this is how I do it') and faith ('trust me, I'm a teaching expert'). This differs from an approach that would look to see whether we can detect any common themes in the behaviours of the teachers of those learners who are achieving. Or indeed, whether we can map those recommendations against measures of learning or student progress.

Part of the reason for this of course is that it is very hard to be certain what actually does influence the development of students' learning. Despite a wealth of literature, both opinion and evidence, on cognitive styles, the psychology of learning and how information is processed and activated in learning situations, there is still a leap of faith required to be sure of the extent to which teachers can positively influence that learning journey. Transfer into clinical practice and impact on patient care are long-term outcomes of teaching in clinical settings and many factors can have an effect along the way. The link between our activities as teachers, and practitioner competence may seem too tenuous. In addition it is likely that for some bright, motivated students learning will occur whatever the teacher does.

However as long ago as 1963, a model of school learning proposed that given time and *good teaching* almost all pupils will be able to master what they are being asked to learn. The concept of mastery learning, has since been somewhat displaced by other theories of teaching and learning. It does however, emphasise the role of the teacher in learning.[1]

On the other side of the coin it is well recognised, at least by learners, that 'bad' teaching can get in the way of learning. It is all too easy to demotivate learners and reduce their confidence and trust in themselves as learners. Inexpertly handled remedial interventions at times of dawning 'conscious incompetence' (perhaps a failed exam or a patient complaint) can reinforce the feeling of worthlessness and a disinclination to persevere with learning. Those moving towards 'unconscious incompetence' from a previous position of expertise, perhaps through ill health or a rapidly changing work environment, also need sensitive guidance from expert teachers and mentors. It is easy to see how we could make things worse rather than better if we are clumsy in our feedback skills as we draw learners' attention to their deficiencies.[2]

Students need guidance to develop study skills. Not all learners will demonstrate, for example, the same degree of self directedness at the same chronological stage in their learning and training or, for any one student, in relation to all subject areas. A 'hands-off' teaching style too early in their development or when content is new or uncertain can leave students all at sea and floundering in a morass of unmet and indeed unrecognised learning needs. In Grow's model of the stages of self direction, which we will return to below, unwary teachers can fall into two traps of mismatch: [2]

1 dependent learners with supervisory-style teaching can result in frustrated learners feeling isolated and lacking in direction; fearful of the freedom they are not ready for

2 teaching self directed learners with a coaching-style of teaching risks learner resentment of the authoritarian teacher.

Educational theories might stress the importance of curriculum alignment or sequencing in teaching or emphasise constructivism or discovery learning. Others contrast teachers as managers of learning with their being involved in direction of students. Still more are based on an understanding that teachers are best employed as facilitators of learning. Whichever we subscribe to in a given situation we can see that teachers clearly have a role in student progress.

It would seem less than useful for a teacher to stand by and leave [a learner] alone in his enquiries, hoping that something will happen.[3]

Some of the early experiments with implementing a problem based learning approach to medical undergraduate curricula, may have unwittingly discovered just that.

There are some basic principles, derived predominantly from expert opinion but also from outcomes based evaluation, that tend to be repeated as elements of effective teaching:

• set clear goals and expected outcomes
• provide adequate supervision and assessment against these goals
• provide meaningful feedback
• show concern for students' progress.

Over the past 25 years, work has been done on these areas to link students' opinions about the presence or absence of these factors in their teachers with subsequent development of clinical skills.[4] Such work however tends to be concentrated on 'what to do' rather than 'how to do it'. Developing competency as expert teachers requires us to analyse and reflect on *how* we carry out tasks.

Entwistle points out that we should be on our guard against an expectation that there will be a view of education that delivers a panacea in all teaching and learning situations.[1] Many descriptions of effective teaching, proposed to help the development of teachers, may in fact be an expression of the writer's own preferred learning styles and understanding of how learning occurs. In addition, sometimes such advice appears to be plucked out of the air rather than grounded in theories about learning and learners.

We are familiar with the need to incorporate learner difference in teaching. Work by Honey and Mumford amongst others has drawn attention to the importance of matching learning opportunities provided by the teacher, with the preferred learning styles of the learner. [5] In teaching practice we now routinely spend time determining our learners' preferences. In longitudinal relationships, such as between registrar and trainer in vocational training for general practice this can be straightforward. But we can also attempt to provide teaching and learning activities likely to appeal to different types of learners even when their learning styles are not known to us, such as in one-off teaching situations.

However in the teacher-learner dyad, learner difference is only one variable. Effective teachers are adaptable and flexible in providing variety in their teaching activities. They aim to match their manipulation of the teaching and learning environment to the needs of the learner. But we also believe that teachers should know what type of activities they are most effective at delivering. This book aims to help healthcare teachers reflect on their teaching practice. You should consider how you can implement what is known about best practice in teaching and how you can maximise the advantage to be gained from playing to your own innate strengths and characteristics as teachers. After all, just as mismatched learning styles can cause dysfunctional learning situations, one of the causes of stress in teachers, can be an incongruence between the type of activities they are good at carrying out and external expectations of 'good teaching'.

## Recent developments in NHS healthcare settings in the UK

The impact of continuing changes in, and modernisation of, healthcare is being felt in training and education. The need for high quality teaching staff was reinforced by commitments to education and training in the NHS Plan which emphasised continuous professional development, lifelong learning, increasing training commissions for doctors, nurses and allied health professions, interprofessional learning and working, and preparation of students and staff for new roles and new ways of working.[6]

The importance of developing a learning culture in the NHS has been recognised as to enable skill mix, sharing of good practice and the capacity to learn from errors. Learning is linked with the implementation of good clinical governance strategies.

In August 2004 the requirements of the European Working Time Directive for doctors and dentists in training were implemented. With this change came significant changes in patterns of service delivery which impact on time available for teaching and training. These changes extend the need to ensure that we have teaching staff with flexibility, as well as appropriate qualifications, experience and commitment to deliver education and training to support contemporary healthcare. They also require more robust arrangements for mentorship and feedback to teachers about their abilities and strengths with resultant benefits for students and the student experience.

The role of the healthcare professional as teacher is increasingly recognised as:

> A core professional activity, that cannot be left to chance, aptitude or inclination.[7]

There have been attempts to formally define what makes an effective teacher in the healthcare professions. For doctors, the General Medical Council (GMC) [8] and the Medical Royal Colleges have described the roles, qualities and skills of a doctor who is a competent teacher. Every doctor who is formally appointed to provide clinical or educational supervision for a doctor in training or who undertakes to provide clinical training or supervision for medical students, should demonstrate the following personal and professional attributes:

- a commitment to the professional guidance in *Good Medical Practice* from the GMC[8]
- an enthusiasm for his/her specialty
- a personal commitment to teaching and learning
- sensitivity and responsiveness to the educational needs of students and junior doctors
- the capacity to promote development of the required professional attitudes and values
- an understanding of the principles of education as applied to medicine
- an understanding of research method
- practical teaching skills
- a willingness to develop both as a doctor and as a teacher
- a commitment to audit and peer review of his/her teaching
- the ability to use formative assessment for the benefit of the student/trainee
- the ability to carry out formal appraisal of medical students progress/the performance of the trainee as a practising doctor.

For nurses and midwives there are few practitioners not in some way involved in the training and supervision of others and increasingly these roles are part of their contract of employment. The United Kingdom Central Council for Nursing, Midwifery and Health Visiting (UKCC)'s advisory standards for mentors are: [9]

Effective mentors will develop:

- communication and working relationships enabling:
  - the development of effective relationships based on mutual trust and respect
  - an understanding of how students integrate into practice settings and assisting with this process
  - the provision of ongoing and constructive support for students

- skills of facilitation of learning in order to:
  - demonstrate sufficient knowledge of the students' programme to identify current learning needs
  - demonstrate strategies which will assist with the integration of learning from practice and educational settings
  - create and develop opportunities for students to identify and undertake experiences to meet their learning needs
- skills of assessment in order to:
  - demonstrate a good understanding of assessment and ability to assess
  - implement approved assessment procedures
- skills as a role model in order to:
  - demonstrate effective relationships with patients and clients
  - contribute to the development of an environment in which effective practice is fostered, implemented, evaluated and disseminated
  - assess and manage clinical developments to ensure safe and effective care
- ability to create an environment for learning in order to:
  - ensure effective learning experiences and the opportunity to achieve learning outcomes for students
  - implement strategies for quality assurance and quality audit
- a knowledge base in order to identify, apply and disseminate research findings within the area of practice
- skills to be able to contribute to the development and/or review of courses.

Similarly Wall and McAleer identified the core content for the clinical teaching role by asking consultants and junior hospital doctors what they thought the curriculum should be for teaching medical teachers.[10] In addition Harden has listed the twelve roles of the medical teacher.[11]

Thus, there exists a movement to define what it is that a healthcare teacher does. But what about how they do it?

Hesketh *et al* outlined a framework for developing excellence as a clinical educator that categorises activity into performance of tasks (doing the right thing), approach to tasks (doing the thing right) and professionalism (the right person doing it.).[12] (For more on this model, see also Chapter 3.)

In a discussion of standards for medical educators, Purcell and Lloyd-Jones consider this framework alongside an examination of very different earlier work on the scholarship of teaching model.[7] They conclude that sometimes we can only define good teaching as what a good teacher does. Context and application have much to do with what standards we will aspire to.

This implies that the ability to adapt teaching to the learning style of the current learners, needs also to be combined with an ability to match teaching with other aspects such as the levels of expertise of the learner, a consideration of whether theoretical or practical educational material is being taught and the purpose and context of learning. This adaptability is a key skill of a flexible teacher and is demonstrated as differences in *teaching style*; the way in which teaching tasks are chosen and carried out. Teachers vary in their preference for one or another style of teaching, just as learners demonstrate differences in learning styles. Just as learners can enhance their learning through application of different learning styles in different situations, even those that they are less comfortable with, so too with teachers and teaching style.

Teaching style has been defined by Kathleen Butler as:[13]

> A set of attitudes and actions that open a formal and informal world of learning to the student. It is a subtle force that influences access to learning and teaching by establishing perimeters around acceptable learning procedures, processes and products. It is the powerful force of the teacher's attitude to the student as well as the instructional activities used by the teacher and it shapes the learning teaching experience.

When Kolb described four learning environments, he was setting the scene for our understanding of the impact of teaching styles as well. As Kaufman *et al* point out, Kolb stated that the roles and actions of teachers are dependent on the particular learning context. [14] So we can see that the flow of influence goes in both directions; teachers and learners both contribute to the development of, and are moulded by, the educational environment.

Kolb's four environments are affectively-orientated (feeling); symbolically-orientated (thinking); perceptually-orientated (watching) and behaviourally-orientated (doing).[15] In the affectively-orientated environment, teachers act as role models and relate to learners as equals or 'friendly advisors'. Input to the learners is delivered quickly and is tailored to meet individual needs and objectives. In the symbolically-orientated environment the teacher is accepted as a body of knowledge as well as timekeeper, task master and enforcer of events in order for the learner to reach a solution or goal. The teacher provides guidelines on terminology and rules. In the perceptually-orientated environment, teachers act as 'process facilitators' and there is an emphasis on process rather than solution, and finally in Kolb's understanding of a behaviourally-orientated environment, teachers act as mentors and give counsel.

Teachers actively create, develop and maintain a particular environment by their actions (and we believe they should do this consciously and with insight into what they are doing). Learners, expecting one environment or another because of context, content, cognitive or learning styles, will perpetuate this driver by valuing it as 'good teaching' when they find it.

From Grow's work on self directedness in learning we can already start to see, in Table 1.1, what the content of four teaching styles might look like. [2]

## The development of teaching styles

So what influences which teaching style a teacher adopts? There is some evidence that choice of teaching style is one facet of a teacher's general view about the purposes of education. We can describe two categories of teachers, formal and informal. Formal teachers see their role in terms of the dominance of outcomes such as examination results, demonstration of predetermined competencies and vocational training. These teachers favour a structured approach. Informal teachers stress learners' enjoyment of education and opportunities for self-expression and tend to favour discovery learning. These

**Table 1.1** Adaptation of Grow's stages of self directedness model to show teaching styles.

| Student | Teacher | Task | Teaching activity | Teaching style |
|---------|---------|------|-------------------|----------------|
| Dependent | Authority Coach | Transmission of facts e.g. basic life support | Coaching with immediate feedback Drill Informational lecture | Standing at the front of the class Talking about facts Demonstrating best practice Addressing external targets |
| Interested | Motivator Guide | Processing and application of information e.g. learning the skills of clinical examination | Inspiring lecture plus guided discussion Goal-setting and learning strategies | Talking about how to learn Socratic questioning Providing domain specific knowledge |
| Involved | Facilitator | Development of values e.g. of healthcare ethics and awareness of professional standards | Discussion facilitated by teacher who participates as equal Seminar Group projects | Emotions to the fore Comfortable with the informal curriculum Heuristic style |
| Self directed | Consultant Delegator | Exploration of new territory such as in workplace-based action research | Dissertation Individual work or self-directed study-group | Focusing on developing educational environment Light-touch Intervention in response to request |

two types of teaching tend to map against an understanding of learning strategy that can also be used to suggest that learners tend to be either holists (in at the deep end) or serialists (step by step).

A formal teacher, if asked to identify how to measure an effective teacher, might be inclined to list classroom attributes such as orderliness, adherence to rules and student attentiveness, and stress the importance of knowledge base, preparation of lesson plans and handouts and clarity in setting objectives.

An informal teacher asked the same question might tend to list student attributes such as spontaneity of students' responses, enthusiasm in learners, individuality of contribution.

**Table 1.2** Paradigms of education.

| Paradigm | Curriculum | Purpose of education |
| --- | --- | --- |
| 1 The cultural-transmission code | Content | Transfer |
| 2 The professional accountability code | Process | Instrumental |
| 3 The learner centred code | Process | Development |

We can identify three paradigms of education in Table 1.2 that help further define the link between teaching style and understanding of the purpose of education.

In the first paradigm, teachers who are following a cultural-transmission code will set great store by the comprehensiveness of the supply of information and 'expertness' in delivery and judge a good outcome to be the degree of transfer and retention of information from the teacher to the learner. An effective teaching style here will include an authoritative manner, clarity of presentation perhaps including provision of handouts and coherent alignment of objective setting, teaching activities and assessment of learning.

In the second type of teaching described in Table 1.2, the aim is to develop a process, a skill or behaviour, that can be translated into a clinical setting. Teaching will be judged effective if there is expert demonstration of either the required skill itself or a proxy skill that requires the same competence, opportunity to practice and accurate and immediate feedback on performance. Student learning is measured by mastery of the skill which can include adaptive learning demonstrating discrimination about when the skill should be applied.

In type three teaching listed in Table 1.2, the teaching and learning activity might bear no resemblance to the required competence that the teacher aims to develop. A teacher using this model of what effective teaching looks like might utilise a style that incorporates attention to the development of a safe environment for learners to experiment, encourage and allow opportunistic or 'accidental' learning and draw on learners' experience to become co-teachers.

Clearly an effective teacher will be able to adapt to any one of the three formats depending on the subject matter and other variables. Flight attendants teaching about emergency exits, or instructors in basic life support are likely to adopt type one. Practical simulator-based sessions aimed at gathering skills such as laparoscopic surgery might be an example of type two. And the use of arts and humanities to develop insight and empathy for patient experience might be an example of type three.

Teachers (or more accurately, researchers in educational theory) have over time described a number of discourses – filters or constructs – to think about teaching and learning. These also help us to refine what we understand to be effective teaching, or how an effective teacher behaves, and how our understanding of a particular educational paradigm can influence our judgement of what constitutes an effective teaching style when we see it.

Consider Table 1.3, which is drawn from some of the thinking by Brian Hodges at the University of Toronto on this subject: [16]

**Table 1.3** The discourses of competence.

| Title of discourse | Measure of competence | Role of teacher | Role of student |
| --- | --- | --- | --- |
| Harrison's textbook | Knowledge | Provider of facts, source of knowledge Explanation of first principles | Memorise facts for recall |
| Miller's pyramid | Performance | Teach skills Provide simulations (practise with scenarios) | Practise and demonstrate skills in performance-based tests |
| Cronbach's alpha | Reliable test score | Preparation of students for assessment (practise with checklists) | Maximise data points in checklist styles assessment |
| Schon's reflective practice | Self assessment by portfolio | Motivator Confessor Mentor | Record reflective writing in portfolio |

Discourse analysis is helpful to consider why there is such fierce debate about what constitutes 'good teaching'. It helps explain that although students can recognise it, and teachers can recognise it, and educational researchers can recognise it, they don't always agree about its presence or absence at any one time. Or about how to measure it. It all depends on what you think education *should be for*.

The problem with a rigid adherence to one or other of these constructs, and an application of a teaching style based on the understanding of that paradigm, is that although we have with each an explicit measure of incompetence, we also have what Brian Hodges calls, 'side effects' – hidden incompetencies,[16] as in Table 1.4.

So we can see that an over-rigid adherence to one or other of these discourses can lead to hidden incompetence in learners; this has implications for our understanding of what constitutes an effective teaching style. We can also see that we need to be clear about what goals we understand the teaching situation to be aimed at, what is to be our measure of success.

For example, if we want safe drivers we need a teaching situation that can lead to competence in performance of certain skills, plus retention of knowledge about rules of the road and also some ability to problem solve in unexpected situations like ice or sudden obstacles on the road. Effective driving instructors thus not only take learner difference into account, but also use varied styles when striving to teach various aspects of the driving tasks – desk-based learning for the Highway Code, simulators for reactions to unexpected events, and road practise to gain confidence and competence.

Healthcare straddles art and science. Whatever our professional background, we understand all of our disciplines to have a strong scientific knowledge base but we also expect a degree of social or behavioural science

**Table 1.4** Hidden incompetencies according to Hodges.

| Title of discourse | Measure of incompetence | Hidden incompetence |
| --- | --- | --- |
| Harrison's textbook | Inability to recall | Cognitive ability to recognise random facts rather than interpret patterns<br>Poor interpersonal behaviours |
| Miller's pyramid | Inability to perform | Inauthentic skills e.g. simulation of empathy |
| Cronbach's alpha | Inability to score highly on checklists or standardised simulations | Inability of assessment tools (e.g. Objective Structured Clinical Examinations (OSCEs)) to capture increasing expertise |
| Schon's reflective practice | Cannot produce convincing analysis of self-efficacy | Cannot identify deficiencies, cannot direct learning due to lack of knowledge |

through which we interpret and apply that knowledge. We might know that certain drugs lower lipid levels, know the biochemical mechanism through which they do that and know that in populations their use can reduce the incidence of heart disease. But we expect practitioners to be able to understand how to take individual patient values into account to see whether a sixth drug, with potential side effects, added to their daily regime is appropriate for them in their context.

So the entrants to our fields will come both from those who have an interest in understanding more about the science base and from those who have an interest in applying it in partnership with patients. One of the mismatches that we sometimes experience between teaching and learning can arise out of this difference. Teaching of basic science often requires a step-wise approach. It depends on facts and knowledge to build up new ideas. Social studies draws more on experience – both of learners and patients – and extrapolation to build new ideas. Field-dependent learners, those who tend to be more informal, may prefer their teachers to be more discursive in their teaching styles. They are at risk of feeling less comfortable with the more convergent, structured approach that we might see in science-based teaching. Similarly field–independent learners, who tend to be more structured in their approach, might be less comfortable with discussion-based or divergent methods.

Flexible teachers not only have to be able to understand and teach in both ways, they need to be able to understand barriers to effective learning that such differences in cognitive styles can raise if not acknowledged.

Even more fundamentally, the choice of style of teaching might usefully be linked to whether a person understands there to be a truth or knowledge 'out there' to be discovered (an ontological approach to education), or the view that we construct our own reality, which is of necessity different for all of us (an epistemological approach). Sometimes the first approach is entirely appropriate and we can test whether a learner knows certain things that we know. In all other situations, learners can be frustrated by our inability as teachers to tell them 'the answer' that they can learn for the exam. Whichever our construct of reality is, just as with our constructs of teaching, we will help our learners more if we can acknowledge the difference. One of the ways our teaching styles can reflect that is in our use of language. We can reflect it in the 'mood' of verbs we use to describe findings, perhaps avoiding the indicative (that affirms or denies) in favour of the subjunctive – the mood that expresses condition, hypothesis, or contingency.

Kathleen Butler has articulated a set of assumptions that might be said to underlie the application of an understanding of the importance of differences in teaching style:[13]

- as a teacher I must understand myself and my goals before I can understand or accept others and their goals
- as a teacher I bring a unique and natural set of qualities that have positive and negative sides – in intent as well as action
- as a teacher, I should not try to fit someone else's model of the competent teacher
- as a teacher I have the power and capacity to do more than teach content, and to aid students on a path of self-discovery
- as a teacher I should use my understanding of the difference in teaching and learning styles to know why I teach as I do and be intentional about my teaching.

This book offers descriptions of, and applications for, different teaching styles. We do this because we believe that different situations require different interventions from teachers. But we also understand that some teachers prefer some teaching styles, or believe themselves to be better at one rather than another, or even that one style is in and of itself 'better teaching' than another. Just as we encourage our students to complete a full journey round the experiential learning cycle to maximise their learning, we would urge teachers to stop and think about their preferred teaching styles. All teachers should consider how they might develop other styles, for different situations, to the benefit of their learners.

# References

1　Entwistle NJ. *Styles of Learning and Teaching*. London: David Fulton Publishers; 1988.

2　Bennett SN. *Teaching Styles and Pupil Progress*. London: Open Books; 1976.

3　Mohanna K, Wall D, Chambers R. *Teaching Made Easy: a manual for health professionals*. 2nd ed. Oxford: Radcliffe Medical Press; 2004.

4　Petzel RA, Harris IB, Masler DS. The empirical validation of clinical teaching strategies. *Eval Health Prof*. 1922; **5,4**: 499–508.

5　Honey P, Mumford A. *Using Your Learning Styles*. Maidenhead: Peter Honey Publications; 1986.

6    Department of Health. *The NHS Plan: a plan for investment, a plan for reform*. London: DH; 2000.

7    Purcell N, Lloyd-Jones G. Standards for medical educators. *Med Educ*. 2003; **37**: 149–54.

8    General Medical Council. *Good Medical Practice*. London: General Medical Council; 2006.

9    The United Kingdom Central Council for Nursing, Midwifery and Health Visiting (UKCC). *Standards for the Preparation of Teachers of Nursing, Midwifery and Health Visiting*. London: UKCC; 2000.

10   Wall D, McAleer S. Teaching the consultant teachers: identifying the core content. *Med Educ*. 2000; **34**: 131–8.

11   Harden R, Crosby JR. *The good teacher is more than a lecturer: the twelve roles of the teacher*. AMEE Education Guide 20. Centre for Medical Education, Dundee; 2000.

12   Hesketh EA, Bagnall G, Buckley EG, *et al*. A framework for developing excellence as a clinical educator. *Med Educ*. 2001; **35**: 555–64.

13   Butler KA. *Learning and Teaching Style: in theory and practice*. Connecticut: The Learner's Dimension; 1984.

14   Kaufman DM, Mann KV, Jennett PA. *Teaching and learning in medical education: how theory can inform practice*. Edinburgh: ASME; 2000.

15   Kolb DA. *Experiential Learning: experience as the source of learning and development*. Englewood Cliffs (NJ): Prentice Hall; 1984.

16   Hodges B. University of Toronto Wilson Centre for Research in Education, Toronto, Canada. Personal communication, AMEE 2006, Genoa, Italy.

# Chapter 2

# Determining your teaching style

*David Wall*

## Introduction

This chapter is in two parts. We start with an account of why we set out to study teaching styles, how we carried out and analysed a questionnaire survey, the results we got and the implications from our work allowing us to construct a tool to enable teaching style to be determined. The second part contains the Staffordshire Evaluation of Teaching Styles (SETS) tool itself so that you can find our your own preferred learning style.

One of our initial aims was to help to cultivate flexibility in novice teachers. Then, help them to understand that they may have to work on improving their least preferred teaching styles in order to be a more flexible learner-centred teacher, and adapt their teaching style to their audience of learners.

Using factor analysis (which is explained in greater depth, with the description of our work, in the Appendix at the end of this book), we found that various professional groups clustered around different factors. This means that it is possible to detect differences in teaching styles that seem to vary with professional groups. This might reflect previous teaching in certain professional groups that moulds both the actions of teachers and also their expectations of what constitutes an effective teaching style.

This chapter includes a brief outline of each of the six teaching styles we have described. These will be expanded in further chapters, where we will give much more detailed descriptions and lots of helpful suggestions on how to be really effective in a preferred style, and how to improve a least preferred style.

## Part 1

### Why we did the study

We wondered if people's teaching styles were distinct and could be measured. We know that there is much work in the educational literature on learning styles. This includes the work of Kolb with his four step learning cycle, using the four roles of converger, diverger, assimilator and accommodator.[1] Honey and Mumford took this further as the four corresponding styles of activist, reflector, theorist and pragmatist.[2] Many of you will have already done this questionnaire on one or more occasions. In addition there are many other concepts in relation to learning styles, including the work of Pask on serialist and holist thinkers,[3] the work of Fleming on the VARK styles (visual, aural, read/write and kinaesthetic)[4] and the work on multiple intelligences by Gardner.[5]

However, this may not be the whole picture. The teacher, the organisations in which we work, society and others are key stakeholders in the business of teaching and learning. Bleakley has suggested that no single theory about learners has enough explanatory power to inform and explain the complex range of practices found in medicine.[6] Bleakley held that the activity theory model[7] with rules, stakeholders and division of labour may be a helpful model in which to conceptualise a medical education model, rather than just looking at the learners. The model, represented in Figure 2.1 shows how all six of the areas connect and are influenced by the other areas.

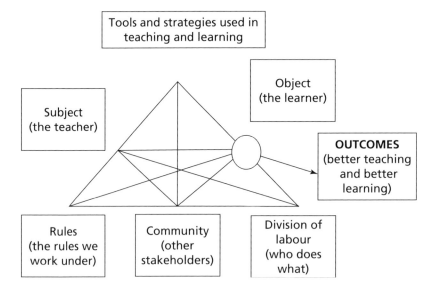

**Figure 2.1** The activity theory model applied to medical education.

We wanted to find a way to identify and analyse teaching styles, and to help novice teachers develop their teaching strategies. We wished to help them find out about their preferred styles and other styles they were less comfortable with using. We wanted to help them think about dysfunctional situations where a mismatch of teaching and learning styles may be the problem, and to be able to analyse their actions and reactions using significant event analysis.

Our work enabled us to test out a large series of aspects of teaching that we had initially derived from a study of the educational literature. We analysed them looking for patterns and associations. Our exploratory factor analysis (see Appendix page 117) showed six themes, which were clearly identifiable with different teaching styles. We developed these six themes into our six teaching styles using free text descriptors from the four key items that most strongly linked to each of the themes. This also turned out to have high face validity.

These six teaching styles are described in much greater detail in the following chapters in this book but short descriptions of each are as follows:

1  **The all-round flexible and adaptable teacher.** This teacher can use lots of different skills, can teach both peers and juniors, and is very aware of the whole environment in relation to teaching and the learners
2  **The student-centred, sensitive teacher.** This teacher is very student-centred, teaches in small groups, with emotions to the fore, using role play and drama, and is not comfortable doing straight presentations
3  **The official curriculum teacher.** This teacher is very well prepared as a teacher, accredited, aware of and teaches to the formal curriculum and follows external targets for teaching
4  **The straight facts no nonsense teacher.** This teacher likes to teach the clear facts, with straight talking, concentrating on specific skills, and much prefers not to be involved with multi-professional teaching and learning
5  **The big conference teacher.** This teacher likes nothing better than to stand up in front of a big audience but not sitting in groups or one to one teaching
6  **The one-off teacher.** This teacher likes to deliver small self contained bits of teaching, on a one to one basis, with no props to help and no follow up.

The outcome of our research was the development of a self evaluation questionnaire, which appears as part two of this chapter. There is also a scoring sheet. Together these allow teachers to derive a personal score for each style and ascertain their strongest preferences. You can visualise the combination of your teaching style as the Staffordshire Hexagon, see page 21.

As an illustration, we have plotted two examples of the Staffordshire Hexagon in Figures 2.2 and 2.3.

In Figure 2.2 the teacher shows a preference to be an all-round adaptable and flexible teacher, in contrast to the pattern of the teacher in Figure 2.3, where the pattern is quite different, with a predominance to be a big conference teacher, with higher scores for the one-off teacher as well as the straight facts no nonsense teacher.

## Conclusions

This chapter, with more detail in the Appendix to the book, tells the story of how we developed the teaching styles project, from the original literature, the questionnaire to determine the preferred teaching styles, how we achieved six styles and their descriptors, and then how we developed the self evaluation

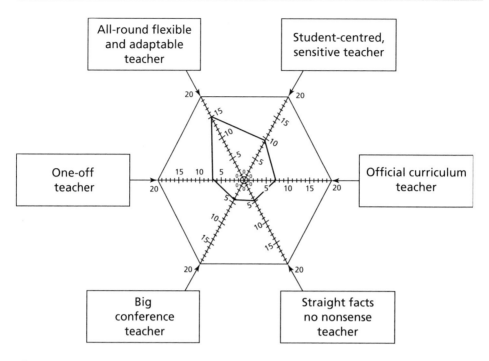

**Figure 2.2** The Staffordshire Hexagon with one style pattern.

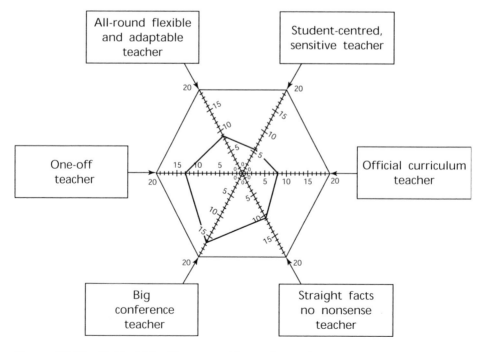

**Figure 2.3** The Staffordshire Hexagon with another style pattern.

questionnaire to score these styles for individual teachers. Further work is in progress to develop and delineate these areas of teaching styles.

The following chapters describe each of the six teaching styles in much greater detail, including tips and advice on how to maximise your preferred teaching style, using educational concepts, maps and models and theoretical frameworks, and also how to improve your least preferred styles. Hopefully you will be able to use the self evaluation questionnaire to see what your own preferred styles are. We hope that as well as concentrating on your preferred styles, you will also take some time to try to develop your other, least preferred styles as well, to help you become more flexible in your approach to teaching.

# Part 2

*The self evaluation tool: the Staffordshire Evaluation of Teaching Styles (SETS).* ©Reproduced with permission of Kay Mohanna, Ruth Chambers, David Wall, Staffordshire University 2007; r.chambers@staffs.ac.uk

This short questionnaire, the SETS, will help you to find out about your preferred teaching styles.

Please rate how much you agree with each of the statements below on the five point scale. Remember that 1 is not agreeing at all through to 5 which is very strongly agree. So the more you agree, the higher the score. Once you have scored yourself, then you will be able to map out your preferred teaching styles using the scoring grid that follows on page 19 and put these scores into the six teaching styles diagram (see Figure 2.4).

|     |                                                                                          | not agree at all | | | strongly agree | |
| --- | ---------------------------------------------------------------------------------------- | --- | --- | --- | --- | --- |
| Q1  | I vary my approach depending on my audience                                              | 1 | 2 | 3 | 4 | 5 |
| Q2  | I am less comfortable giving straight presentations than teaching through games and exercises | 1 | 2 | 3 | 4 | 5 |
| Q3  | I prefer to teach through games to relay learning                                        | 1 | 2 | 3 | 4 | 5 |
| Q4  | I like having external targets to determine the course of learning                       | 1 | 2 | 3 | 4 | 5 |
| Q5  | I prefer teaching sessions that are self-contained with no follow-up                     | 1 | 2 | 3 | 4 | 5 |
| Q6  | Props often detract from a talk                                                          | 1 | 2 | 3 | 4 | 5 |
| Q7  | I am comfortable addressing large audiences                                              | 1 | 2 | 3 | 4 | 5 |
| Q8  | Preparation for my teaching focuses on me and my role                                    | 1 | 2 | 3 | 4 | 5 |

| | | | | | | |
|---|---|---|---|---|---|---|
| Q9 | I am usually standing up when I teach | 1 | 2 | 3 | 4 | 5 |
| Q10 | The best teaching sessions convey straight facts in a clear way | 1 | 2 | 3 | 4 | 5 |
| Q11 | I avoid being distracted from running sessions the way I plan to run them | 1 | 2 | 3 | 4 | 5 |
| Q12 | I am happy teaching general skills | 1 | 2 | 3 | 4 | 5 |
| Q13 | I put no value on being formally employed as a teacher | 1 | 2 | 3 | 4 | 5 |
| Q14 | I dislike one to one teaching | 1 | 2 | 3 | 4 | 5 |
| Q15 | I am consistent in delivery of a topic, whatever the audience | 1 | 2 | 3 | 4 | 5 |
| Q16 | I like to give students opportunity to explore how to learn | 1 | 2 | 3 | 4 | 5 |
| Q17 | I have developed my own style as a teacher | 1 | 2 | 3 | 4 | 5 |
| Q18 | I prefer one to one teaching | 1 | 2 | 3 | 4 | 5 |
| Q19 | Eliciting emotions through role play or drama is a valuable aspect of teaching | 1 | 2 | 3 | 4 | 5 |
| Q20 | I am comfortable using humour in my teaching | 1 | 2 | 3 | 4 | 5 |
| Q21 | I rarely sit down when with students | 1 | 2 | 3 | 4 | 5 |
| Q22 | It is important to me that my teaching is accredited by an official body | 1 | 2 | 3 | 4 | 5 |
| Q23 | I am uncomfortable when I have multi-professional groups of learners to teach | 1 | 2 | 3 | 4 | 5 |
| Q24 | I am at my best when organising my teaching to fit an external curriculum or organisational structure | 1 | 2 | 3 | 4 | 5 |

## The Scoring Grid for the SETS Tool

Once you have filled in your own scores for all of the 24 questions on the SETS questionnaire, you will need to transfer the score for each question into the six teaching styles on page 20. The questions on the SETS have been randomly allocated on the questionnaire, so it is important that you allocate the marks correctly to each teaching style.

| Question | Style One | Style Two | Style Three | Style Four | Style Five | Style Six |
|----------|-----------|-----------|-------------|------------|------------|-----------|
| **Q1** | Q1 = 4 | | | | | |
| **Q2** | | Q2 = 3 | | | | |
| **Q3** | | Q3 = 4 | | | | |
| **Q4** | | | Q4 = 2 | | | |
| **Q5** | | | | | | Q5 = 2 |
| **Q6** | | | | | | Q6 = 2 |
| **Q7** | | | | | Q7 = 3 | |
| **Q8** | | | Q8 = 4 | | | |
| **Q9** | | | | | Q9 = 3 | |
| **Q10** | | | | Q10 = 4 | | |
| **Q11** | | | | Q11 = 3 | | |
| **Q12** | Q12 = 4 | | | | | |
| **Q13** | | | | | | Q13 = 2 |
| **Q14** | | | | | Q14 = 2 | |
| **Q15** | | | | Q15 = 3 | | |
| **Q16** | | Q16 = 4 | | | | |
| **Q17** | Q17 = 4 | | | | | |
| **Q18** | | | | | | Q18 = 3 |
| **Q19** | | Q19 = 3 | | | | |
| **Q20** | Q20 = 3 | | | | | |
| **Q21** | | | | | Q21 = 2 | |
| **Q22** | | | Q22 = 3 | | | |
| **Q23** | | | | Q23 = 3 | | |
| **Q24** | | | Q24 = 3 | | | |
| *TOTALS* | 15 | 14 | 12 | 13 | 10 | 9 |

Please fill in your score for each of the questions in the correct boxes on page 19, then add the columns up to obtain your score for each of the six teaching styles (out of a maximum of 20 marks).

Next, please fill in your scores obtained from the chart totals above, into the six boxes against each of the teaching styles below.

**Style One:** The all-round flexible and adaptable teacher

This teacher can use lots of different skills, can teach both peers and juniors, and is very aware of the whole environment both in teaching and of the learners.

**Style Two:** The student-centred, sensitive teacher

This teacher is very student-centred, teaches in small groups, with emotions to the fore, using role play and drama, and is not comfortable doing straight presentations.

**Style Three:** The official curriculum teacher

This teacher is very well prepared as a teacher, accredited, is very aware of and teaches to the formal curriculum and follows external targets for teaching.

**Style Four:** The straight facts no nonsense teacher

This teacher likes to teach the clear facts, with straight talking, concentrating on specific skills, and much prefers not to be involved with multi-disciplinary teaching and learning.

**Style Five:** The big conference teacher

This teacher likes nothing better than to stand up in front of a big audience. This teacher does not like sitting in groups or one to one teaching.

**Style Six**: The one-off teacher

This teacher likes to deliver small self-contained bits of teaching, on a one to one basis, with no props to help and no follow up.

So now you have the scores out of 20 for your own self evaluation of your preferred teaching styles. Now please go on to Figure 2.4, the Staffordshire Hexagon: a diagrammatic representation of your preferred teaching styles.

Please take the marks from the six boxes and put a cross along each of the six axes to represent your score in each of the six teaching styles. You may wish to join up the crosses to produce a shape of your own combination of styles.

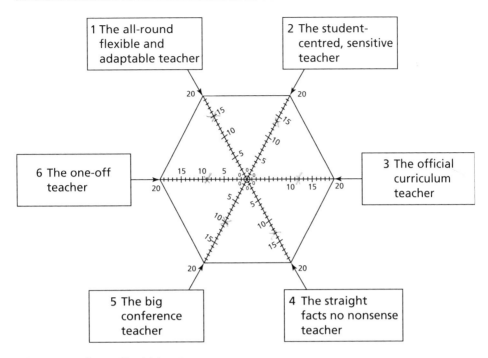

**Figure 2.4** The Staffordshire Hexagon.

# References

1    Kolb DA. *Experiential Learning: experience as the source of learning and development.* Englewood Cliffs (NJ): Prentice Hall; 1984.

2.   Honey P, Mumford A. *Using Your Learning Styles.* Maidenhead: Peter Honey Publications; 1986.

3.   Pask G. Styles and strategies of learning. *Brit J Educ Psychol.* 1976; **46**: 128–48.

4.   Fleming ND. *Teaching and learning styles: VARK strategies.* Christchurch, NZ: Neil Fleming; 2001.

5.   Gardner H. *Multiple Intelligences after 20 years.* Paper presented at the American Educational Research Association, Chicago, Illinois, USA, on 21 April 2003. At http://pzweb.harvard.edu/PIs/HG_MI_after_20_years.pdf (accessed 18 December 2006).

6.   Bleakley A. Broadening conceptions of learning in medical education: the message from teamworking. *Med Educ.* 2006; **40**: 150–7.

7.   Cole M, Engeström, Y. A cultural-historical approach to distributed cognition. In: Salomon G, editor. *Distributed Cognitions.* Cambridge: Cambridge University Press; 1993. 1–46.

# Chapter 3

# The all-round flexible and adaptable teacher

*Kay Mohanna*

Through our work with expert teachers we have defined the all-round flexible teacher thus:

> This teacher can use lots of different skills effectively, can teach both peers and juniors, and is very aware of the way that the whole environment affects both teachers and learners.

## What does this style mean?

Good teachers recognise that learners differ. We all come to learning with different experiences and pre-existing expertise, different levels of motivation and preferred ways of learning. Learners also have an understanding of what teaching and learning is, based on previous instructional experiences and hence they have expectations of their teacher. This will colour how they enter into and respond in a new learning situation. The skill of being a great teacher is in knowing how to respond to learners in ways that effectively address the differences between them and to be able to facilitate learning in a variety of ways that also takes into account differences in subject matter and setting.

For example, based on work by Marton and Saljo, we can recognise two approaches to learning that will serve in different settings: *deep* and *surface*.[1] These approaches depend on a student's understanding of learning, that can be described in five stages:

1  learning is an increase in knowledge: something done to the learner by the teacher
2  learning is memorising: the student actively memorises information but does not transform it in any way
3  learning is the acquisition of facts or procedures to be used: skills or formulae for example are learnt to be used at a later date but there is still no transforming of information
4  learning is making sense: the student will make an active search for abstract meaning in the process of learning

5 learning is understanding reality: a personally meaningful process that enables the world to be perceived differently.

Students who understand learning at a surface level, levels 1–3, will have trouble comprehending a deep approach and are unlikely to take a deep approach to learning. They will always adopt a surface approach because of their understanding of what learning is (acquisition of knowledge) and their experience of previous teaching. Those who have an understanding of the deeper levels 4 and 5 however, can take either a deep or surface approach depending on the task.

Not surprisingly there is a relationship between the understanding of learning and expectations of teaching. Learners in the reproducing group, 1–3, expect teaching to be closed, i.e. teachers select the content, present it to the student and then test to see if it has 'stuck'. Learners in the making sense group, 4 and 5, feel that teaching should be 'open', i.e. the learner functions independently with the facilitation by the teacher.

Often learners are in the reproducing group at levels 1–3 simply because they have only been exposed to 'closed' teaching, especially that involved in exam preparation. Students can become more sophisticated as learners if they experience a more 'open' learning environment. There is a considerable amount of evidence that assessment systems dominate what students are orientated towards in their learning. Development of tasks that make different demands on students requiring them to learn at a deeper level can develop their understanding of what learning is and hence their choices in a learning situation.

This draws on a third approach to learning, which Biggs defined as the strategic or 'achievement approach.[2] Here, the emphasis is on organising learning specifically to pass assessments. A deep learner may adopt some of the strategies of the surface learner to meet the requirements of the test. So 'deep' or 'surface' approaches are not fixed. Strategic learners can recognise the difference.

Characteristics of teaching environments that could foster a *surface* approach to learning include:

- heavy workload
- relatively high class contact hours
- excessive amount of course material
- lack of opportunity to pursue subjects in depth
- lack of choice over subjects and a lack of choice over methods of study
- a threatening and anxiety provoking assessment system.

In addition, characteristics of teaching that could foster a *deep* approach to learning have been identified by Biggs:

- motivational content: who owns the agenda of the teaching? Students learn best when they understand the importance of what they are learning and are involved in selecting what is learnt and planning how this learning will take place
- learner activity: active participation enables links to be made between new concepts and past learning. Activity alone however is insufficient. It must

be planned, reflected upon, processed and integrated with abstract concepts (the learning cycle)
- interaction with others. It can be easier to negotiate meaning and to manipulate ideas with others than alone
- well structured knowledge base. If a student is to integrate new learning with previous knowledge there must be order and structure to the learning.

**Table 3.1** What the clinician as teacher is able to do: 'doing the right thing'.

| Activity | How flexible are you in encouraging deep learning? |
| --- | --- |
| Teach large and small groups | Are you comfortable selecting from a variety of different teaching formats to match the requirements of the learning objectives? |
| | When did you last attend as a learner to develop your competence in alternative teaching strategies? |
| Teach in a clinical setting | Do you provide examples from practice and problem based learning scenarios grounded in real life to provide a context to interpretation and retention of complex information? |
| | Do you encourage the involvement of patients in teaching as partners in the educational process? |
| Facilitate and manage learning | Can you help learners effectively diagnose their own learning needs and devise targeted learning to fill gaps?<br>Are you able to seek and respond to learner feedback? |
| | Do you have a structured approach to interpreting and addressing potential barriers to learning? |
| Plan learning | Do you understand and apply the basic principles of curriculum design? |
| | Have you considered the order, structure and delivery of what is to be learnt and how your subject fits with what else is to be learnt? |
| Develop and work with learning resources | Do you understand the principles of instructional media design, including the range of different ways in which learners prefer to receive and process information? |
| Assess trainees | Have you been trained in the application of current assessment tools in your discipline? |
| | Do you understand what makes an assessment valid and reliable and what the pitfalls are to avoid in assessment – both formative and summative? |
| | Are you able to align your choice of assessment tool with the educational objectives and with the domain of learning to ensure your assessment tool drives learning in the direction of the required outcomes? |

In the healthcare professions, where it is clearly impossible to operate at level 1–3 and cover the whole subject area, we need to foster a deeper approach to learning in ourselves and our students. Learning should be directed at an understanding of how to find things out, rather than just the acquisition of facts. We can work towards this by attention to how we plan teaching activities, especially assessment tasks.

We referred earlier (see Chapter 1) to the framework for developing excellence as a clinical teacher.[3] This list of tasks, can be useful to analyse our activity, looking for evidence that we are encouraging deep or effective learning. The all-round flexible teacher will demonstrate their understanding of educational theory in the kind of environment he or she promotes. Tables 3.1, 3.2 and 3.3 show some suggestions as to how that might be analysed, in the form of a series of questions around the tasks of a teacher, as divided by Hesketh *et al* into 'what the clinician is able to do', 'how the clinician approaches teaching', and 'the clinician as a professional teacher'.[3]

## Is this style really you?

You may feel after reading through what it takes to be an effective all-round flexible teacher, that you really have one strength and would prefer to play

**Table 3.2** How the clinician approaches teaching: 'doing the thing right'.

| *Approach* | *How do you encourage effective learning?* |
|---|---|
| With understanding of educational principles | How aware are you of important background educational theories and current understanding of how learners learn? |
| With appropriate attitudes, ethical understanding and legal awareness | How do you create a safe environment for learners working in healthcare where they experience illness, death and bereavement? |
| | Do you promote an environment where adverse incident reporting and significant event analysis are effective learning tools? |
| | Do you effectively and respectively involve patients in teaching, both as teachers and resources? |
| With appropriate decision making skills and best evidence based education | How do you use educational theory to plan and develop your teaching interventions? |
| | To what extent do you plan to teach based on 'what I know worked for me' compared to an understanding of learner difference? |
| | What evaluative techniques do you apply to ensure your effectiveness as a teacher? |

**Table 3.3** The clinician as professional teacher: 'the right person doing it'.

| Attribute | How do you encourage effective learning? |
|---|---|
| The role of the teacher within the health service or university | Do you take time to consider yourself as a role model and the influence you have on learners through the hidden curriculum? |
| | Do you take care to minimise the effect of the null curriculum? |
| | What attention do you give to the development of lifelong learning skills to ensure effective and safe professional performance by your learners? |
| | Do you contribute to developing an academic community by networking and sharing best practice? |
| | Do you contribute to the educational literature though research, audit or evaluation with presentation or publication? |
| Personal development with regard to teaching | How up to date are you with advances in the educational literature? |
| | Do you regularly gather, reflect on *and respond* to learner feedback? |
| | Have you participated in peer observation and feedback on your teaching to increase your insight into those attributes you possess that will encourage deep learning? |

to that rather than aspire to be a 'Jack of all Trades'. You may feel that being an effective teacher includes recognising your limitations. Certainly it will take self-awareness, feedback from others, and practice for you to be able to adopt or adapt different teaching styles to match the purpose of the learning you are delivering to the preferences or needs of all trainees or all topics.

However the skill of recognising variation in teaching style is in itself a useful advantage for a teacher. You can use skills of delegation, team work or professional networking to enable to you to call on other sources of expertise as and when needed. You may feel that your particular strengths lie in the organisation of educational events, ensuring a mixture of resources is available for learners. Seminars, one to one tutorials, one-off lectures and round table discussions require different skills of facilitation, and it could be argued that it is unlikely to find all those skills rolled up into one person.

The all-round flexible teacher does however possess one skill we should all aspire to as teachers; the main role of any teacher is to create an educational environment that supports learning. All-round teachers can do this effectively in different contexts, but for those teachers who aspire to be experts in another teaching style, this is still integral to those roles.

## Making the most of this as your preferred style and improving it if it is your least preferred style

The importance of building a conducive educational environment is linked to our aim of engaging the learners in the learning process. For engagement we require motivated learners, who understand the relevance of what they are required to learn and we need to pay attention to the role of learners in the organisation, as well as the content and organisation of curriculum. We need to demonstrate that we value learners as future members of the profession and that we have taken time and trouble to ensure barriers to involvement in education have been minimised.

Effective all-round flexible teachers demonstrate creative, innovative and novel solutions to the practical problems of teaching in clinical settings, which are based on critique of the literature as well as original thought. Whatever your teaching styles though, all teachers should work towards developing a safe learning environment based on the principles of adult learning and incorporating trainee evaluation of the teaching. For those teaching predominantly in one style, either through choice or circumstance, learner and peer feedback will be an important source of insight into how well this aspect of the role is managed and to demonstrate areas for self development. It is important to remember that it is student achievement that is the mark of effective teaching.

The following list of activities has been distilled from various writers, looking at the role of both mentoring and instruction in the clinical setting. We can think about how we promote an effective learning environment in our own setting by considering nine areas (modified from Stuart).[4]

1 Ensure learners feel able to seek help without loss of confidence or self esteem by attending to the way questions are answered and requests for support are handled. In group teaching we enhance this when we avoid ridiculing those asking questions, encourage group members to offer suggested answers, praise new ideas and acknowledge when we ourselves don't have the answer. In one to one clinical situations we develop this when we are available to juniors and have a structured response to mistakes and critical incidents.

2 Foster that feeling of self-confidence with praise and constructive feedback, i.e. feedback that is high in support but high in challenge, robustly identifying areas for development. It helps to give feedback and answer questions by assessing what level of learning is occurring. For example, when a student is moving from exploration to understanding, effective teachers recognise this, avoid frustrating learners and give direct answers to content based questions. When learners are focusing on actions that can be taken, facilitation requires us to move into further development of knowledge and skills which might require practice rather than instruction.

3 Try to build in an element of choice about cases learners are exposed to, topics they research or subjects they can investigate. We can build on incidental learning from almost any topic if we encourage learners to reflect on what they have learnt and transfer important generalisable

concepts into other areas. Self-selection motivates learners to learn as they have identified a learning need.

4 Awareness of the power of role modelling as a way to reinforce desired behaviours.

5 Encourage self-monitoring and evaluation of performance. It is vital that future healthcare professionals are able to assess where they have reached in their learning, assess their own performance and set realistic targets for development.

6 Be prepared to listen to and learn from the experiences learners describe. Rogers suggested that facilitators need to be able to recognise and respond to the emotions learners display, not always an easy task. [5]

7 Give learners time to reflect on what has happened and is happening, promote discussion about patient care and always allow time to debrief following significant events.

8 Allow learners to make mistakes within the limits of patient safety but be aware of the power of the teacher to manipulate events to allow success.

9 Show confidence in the abilities of learners; reinforce the expectation of success.

# References

1   Marton F, Saljo R. Approaches to learning. In: Marton F, Hounsell D, Entwistle N, editors. *The Experience of Learning*. Edinburgh: Scottish Academic Press; 1984.

2   Biggs J, Moore P. *The Process of Learning*. New York: Prentice-Hall; 1993.

3   Hesketh EA, Bagnall G, Buckley EG, *et al*. A framework for developing excellence as a clinical educator. *Med Educ*. 2001; **35**: 555–64.

4   Stuart CC. *Assessment, Supervision and Support in Clinical Practice. A guide for nurses, midwives and other health professionals*. London: Churchill Livingston; 2003.

5   Rogers CR. *Freedom to Learn for the 80s*. Columbus, Ohio: Charles E Merrill; 1983.

# Chapter 4

# The student-centred sensitive teacher

*Kay Mohanna*

> This teacher is very student-centred, teaches in small groups, with emotions to the fore, using role play and drama, and is not comfortable doing straight presentations.

Student-centredness has become very popular in healthcare teaching, perhaps in parallel with moves towards a more explicitly patient-centred NHS. As we aim to develop the skills for future lifelong learning in our learners we often strive to develop their levels of self direction and independence, equipping them with skills to allow them to continue to develop on their own, as well as directing our teaching at their identified areas of need. So, concentrating on the learner either individually or in small groups, seems intuitively to be an appropriate approach. It also has a firm foundation in educational theory, helping to explain how adults learn.

## What does this style mean?

Brookfield described several principles of adult learning that he felt underpinned the development of learners to manage their own learning but also pointed out that for effective learning, students need support and expert facilitation.[1] Learning is a personal activity as individuals make sense of the world from their own perspective and attempt to increase their knowledge and understanding. For that a process of action and reflection is needed – a continuous process of investigation, exploration, action, reflection and further action. Critical reflection brings awareness that alternatives can be presented as challenges to the learner to gather evidence, ask questions and develop a critically aware frame of mind. Without placing the learner at the centre of this model of learning, it is hard to see how this can be effective.

Clearly there is much that new entrants to the healthcare professions will need to know, but a student-centred teacher chooses to help learners acquire new knowledge, skills and attitudes whilst at the same time developing meta-cognitive skills such as in reflective practice, problem solving, team working and critical thinking. These are the same skills that they will need to identify their future deficiencies, carry out self appraisal of performance and personal assessment of learning needs.

In England, the White Paper on the professional regulation of doctors and other health professionals is likely to mean that appraisal – the ability of an established practitioner to self assess, identify and act on current strengths and deficiencies in performance – will move from being a formative to a summative process.[2] Hitherto there has been no obligation on doctors to demonstrate their continuing fitness to practise. In the future the requirement to do so, and to do it partly through the medium of appraisal, will require new approaches to staying up to date and a demonstrable commitment to reflective practice, self directed learning and analysis of performance. Similarly for other healthcare practitioners, the need to *demonstrate* competence is increasingly being linked to educational activities. This brings with it implications for teachers and educational facilitators. Mentoring, appraisal and educational supervision are all processes within this new educational paradigm that will require teachers who are comfortable with this teaching style of student centred sensitivity.

The challenge inherent in this for teachers with a preference for the student-centred teaching style however, is that it is not at all clear that self directiveness is a desirable outcome for all learners. This teaching style does not mean that we all need to become expert at inculcating self directed learning in our trainees. A student-centred approach recognises that not all learners are self directed all the time. Previous experience, expectations of learning and teaching, levels of knowledge and skills, and current topic to be learnt all affect the degree to which a student can be self directed. Brookfield pointed out that self directed learning alone has a less successful outcome than a mix of group activity and self directed endeavour.[1]

Knowles defined self directed learning as a process in which learners take the lead in diagnosing their learning needs, designing learning experiences, locating resources and evaluating their effectiveness as learners.[3] His assumptions about how this happened have led over the years to an increase in the amount of unsupervised learning that is allowed to occur, in the hope that this will lead to learner centred learning. A predicable result is that students can become frustrated as they struggle to find out what it is they need to know and learning can become patchy or opportunistic. Whilst this latter might not matter since a heuristic approach to learning (trial and error) can constantly redefine objectives without predetermined outcomes and plug gaps in knowledge, it is more effective for established practitioners. In this setting effective learning can result from an investigation into areas of interest and curiosity, as much as from problem solving. For new learners however, an effective student-centred approach is likely to need more, not less, facilitation and hands-on teaching.

The key to effective student-centred teaching is an ability to help learners find out what they need to know and to not concentrate overly on things they want to find out or be able to do. This distinction between needs and wants is where expert educational supervision comes in. Needs assessment is a complex process that can be done by individuals on their own but is often enhanced when they go through the process with an educational supervisor or appraiser. Helping learners identify the things they don't know requires you to shine light into the blind spot of their areas of 'unconscious incompetence'. This can be a painful process and requires sensitivity.

We can list a number of different needs assessment exercises, and can see that each will require more or less in the way of facilitation by an educational supervisor or appraiser. The methods of needs assessment for students or new entrants are:

- self assessment against curriculum or course content
- assessment by external assessor, with feedback
- comparison of performance against protocols or guidelines
- task-analysis of role or environment
- feedback from senior colleagues and peers
- reading and reflecting.

And the methods of needs assessment for established practitioners are:

- audit of practice
- assessment of 'risk' in current practice
- critical incident analysis
- analysis of 'uncomfortable moments'
- learning log or diary
- eliciting views of patients
- analysis of population health needs.

| Knowledge | Political awareness | Attitudes | Skills | Aspirations | Context | Legal requirements |
|---|---|---|---|---|---|---|
| clinical | policy | to other disciplines | team working | career | settings | health and safety |
| information | priorities | patient skills | communi-cation | transferable | population | employment |
| resources | fashions | lifelong learning | IT capability | teacher | networks | revalidation |
| experts | change | cultural | organisational development | promotion | organisation's priorities | safe practice |
| best practice | | | specialisms | organisation's mission / vision | team relationships historical service patterns | |
| | | | competent practitioner | | | |

**Stage 1** Where are you now? What are your roles and responsibilities? What do you need to know? What skills do you need?
**Stage 2** Where do you want to be?
**Stage 3** What are your learning needs?
**Stage 4** Prioritise your learning needs.
**Stage 5** What essential and desirable objectives will you focus on?
**Stage 6** What 'tools' (for example skills, resources, qualifications, opportunities) do you have?
**Stage 7** What 'tools' do you need?
**Stage 8** How and when are you going to fulfil your learning objectives?
**Stage 9** How will you know when you have achieved your objectives?

**Figure 4.1** Framework of an educational needs analysis that is relevant to your current service post.

**Table 4.1** Activities to enhance the student-centred sensitive teaching style.

| Strategy | Description | Uses | Drawback |
|---|---|---|---|
| Teaching-learning group | Active, syndicated, self resourced, economical; tutor participates as an equal | To explore demarcated topics particularly skills training, allows comparison and 'benchmarking' of personal progress against that of others in a given topic | Risks individual members dominating and addressing their own learning needs |
| Brainstorming | Capture of ideas | Identification of themes, ideas, new issues or areas for investigation, encourages reflection on current state of knowledge | All ideas risk being given equal prominence unless moderated |
| Action learning | Active, real time, based in practice, iterative | Practical skills including communication and management, addresses current real-life issues, can help learners focus on how to remediate actions that have not worked | May result in learning that is not transferable to other settings, may focus on content rather than process |
| Role play | Experiential, participatory, flexible, analytical | Communication skills, to develop empathy, insight and problem solving, exploration of attitudes | Anxiety provoking and risks harm, needs careful facilitation to deal with exposed feelings and unexpected responses and ensure roles are 'left behind' after the exercise |
| Micro teaching (e.g. videoed) | Personalised, analytical, experiential | Skills training, raised insight and allows feedback on performance | Requires observers and valid and reliable observation tool |
| Trios | Reality based, analytic, experiential | Develop active listening, analysis of differing perspectives, allows 'benchmarking' of self against peers | Risks as for role play, third party observation considered 'true' |
| Syndicate groups | Tutor-less, structured tasks, group as resource | Co-operation, problem solving, shares best practice | Essential learning might not be covered or emphasis shifted |
| Games | Artificial, competitive, non-threatening | Experiential, transferable skills | Can distract from the learning if not well debriefed or moderated |
| Snowballing (pyramiding) | Discussion groups: pairs (e.g. generate a list), fours (classify, prioritise) large group (identify themes, summarise) | Exchange of ideas and values, clarification of individuals' views, importance of consensus | Time consuming |
| Domino (cascade) | Recipients of learning pass it on to others (e.g. teams) | Ensures understanding, builds cooperation and team work, enhances shared group ideals | Risks errors of gaps in understanding being passed on |
| Cross over groups | Active, participatory, discussion and summary | Introductions, cross fertilisation, testing of ideas | Can be repetitive |

The framework in Figure 4.1 can also be used as a basis for facilitators to help learners develop a personal needs assessment.[4] This gives examples of components and topics that might be relevant for a health professional in a particular NHS post assessing their educational needs with respect to their service commitments. Then to reflect on the components of their job and make a comprehensive 9 Stage plan to address their learning needs across the range of their roles.

## Is this style really you?

If you are a student-centred, sensitive teacher quite unlike, for example, the 'straight facts no nonsense teacher', you may be most comfortable helping students to develop in the affective domain – considering attitudes and professional behaviours. In order to achieve this you will design teaching activities that allow learners to discuss and exchange views. At the same time in order to develop knowledge and skills you will design teaching activities around case discussions and consideration of the perspective of all players in a scenario. You may for example develop safe environments where you expect learners to act in role plays. All of these types of activities have particular strengths and drawbacks and require different skills of the facilitator.

Table 4.1 summarises some of the main types of activity that might be used by a teacher comfortable with this teaching style.

Another way of looking at this is that there are several options available to address certain types of educational aim, as listed in Table 4.2. A successful student-centred sensitive teacher will be able to flexibly adopt different strategies.

## Making the most of this as your preferred style

So, having identified your preferred teaching style as the student-centred sensitive style, you will be comfortable and proficient in facilitating learning in a one to one or small group situation.

**Table 4.2** Alternative strategies to achieve student-centred outcomes.

| Educational aim | Methods |
| --- | --- |
| Exploration of attitudes | Problem case analysis, random case analysis, role play, debate, Balint discussions |
| Problem solving | Problem case analysis, brainstorming, buzz groups, critical incident, action learning |
| Communication skills | Micro teaching using videos, role play, trios |
| Learning and study skills | Action learning, teaching-learning group, project learning |
| Presentation skills | Mini-lecture, micro teaching, teaching-learning group |
| New factual learning | Lecture, symposium, seminar, project |

In group situations you will have a working understanding of Bruce Tuckman's 'Forming, Storming, Norming, Performing' team-development model.[5] For this staged model Taraschi has identified specific facilitator behaviours for each of the four group development stages:[6]

1 at the **forming** stage the group is finding an identity and clarifying its role. You may find the group is dependent on you for leadership or facilitation. There will be uneven or tentative participation possibly with quiet defiance. The facilitator role is to model openness, disclosure, and active listening. Useful behaviours will be listening, especially to what is not said. Demonstrate disclosure by expressing your feelings. Be attuned to nonverbal cues that signal apprehension. Be prepared to intervene and ensure objective, goals, and agenda are clear
2 when a group enters the **storming** stage the group is often focused on issues of control with members competing to have their say. At this point it may question your leadership, authority or group rules and you may find verbal or nonverbal resistance. The role of the facilitator is to help the team recognise group dynamics and address conflict positively. You will want to pay particular attention to group dynamics and be specific when describing behaviours. Encourage team members to discuss their feelings as well as their interests versus their positions
3 the third stage is **norming** when the group has settled into a trusting relationship and can recognise and discuss difference. Here the facilitator's role is to uncover unspoken issues and encourage self-critique. You need to be able to immediately point out nonconformance to ground rules, encourage reflection on group process and encourage the full exploration of ideas and inferences
4 the final stage is when the group is **performing** and an interdependence of team members has developed. Your role becomes one of teaching the group to self-facilitate. At this stage you should plan with the group how to share the leadership role and perhaps coach the group itself in facilitation skills.

## Co-facilitating

Another role that we sometimes find ourselves in in small group work is that of co-facilitator. This requires extra skills of cooperation and sensitivity to the position of a colleague. Interestingly the 'rules of engagement' for co-facilitating are less well known.

When two people lead a small group together there is clearly potential to share the work – including both preparation and leading on the day. It also means that there is another person to reflect on what is happening in the group, with the potential to intervene if one facilitator appears to becoming too closely involved in group task, rather than facilitating process. A co-facilitator can give you feedback on how you are doing.

The following ground rules for effective co-facilitation have been developed from the earlier work of Race:[7]

1 decide in advance which model of co-facilitation you are using: is it one lead and one support, is one partner acting as a silent observer, or are you going to share the tasks equally?

2 if you decide that one will 'lead' and the other will be the 'support', discuss at the outset what you actually mean by 'leading' and 'supporting'. For example, if you are the 'lead' what sort of (and how much) intervention do you want from the 'support'? Ensure that participation by group members is not blocked by the tendency of enthusiastic co-facilitators to discuss issues between them. As a rule of thumb, contributions from co-facilitators should be separated by at least one group member's contribution

3 if you elect to have one person as the facilitator proper and the other to be the observer, the observer might feed back their reflections to the facilitator or the group including significant verbatim comments made by participants

4 the second person can act as trouble-shooter for handling difficulties that individual participants are experiencing that do not impact on the rest of the group (e.g., the departure of a participant from the workshop whose child has become ill)

5 the second person can act as scribe for activities that require flipchart recording

6 one person can give the instructions for a syndicate activity and the other can reinforce this on break-out of the groups

7 another type of division of labour is for one person to focus on content issues and for the other to focus on process issues. For example, in a plenary discussion one facilitator takes primary responsibility for the intellectual content and the other takes main responsibility for the other things that are happening within the group. This might include recognising the person who is trying without success to get into the discussion, the person whose twitching foot indicates feelings of irritation, the fact that the session has overrun into scheduled lunch-time and so on.

A recurring theme for seasoned facilitators is to be present and transparent for the group.

> When you facilitate, throw away all of your generalisations and be present to these individuals, this group, here, now.[8]

## Improving this if it is your least preferred style

Effective teachers with a good understanding of educational theory will usually be successfully able to facilitate most types of learning activity in this teaching style. One that is so linked to personality traits such as introversion/extroversion as to make it a particular challenge to teachers for whom this is not their preferred style however, is role play.

Role play, the acting out of simulated situations to practise management techniques or to explore feelings, can be a useful teaching aid. Since it involves observation of us in action in a situation we may have little control over however, it can be perceived as threatening. Not all learners relish the prospect and for some it can be unhelpful and bordering on destructive to confidence and progress, especially if not carefully managed. In addition, people with different learning styles will find role play of varying usefulness.

Not all teachers are comfortable facilitating role play or able to deal with possible unexpected outcomes or unseen consequences. Used well it can be a powerful aid to learning and there is a place for it as we encourage learners to explore their own feelings and those of others in given situations.

Role play works best when there is trust between the participants. The following 'rules' or guidelines for safe and effective role play, make the contract that underlies that feeling of trust explicit.

- Consent: participation is voluntary and all parties must consent to the activity and be able to decline to take part.
- Confidentiality: what happens within the role play remains within the exercise, unless all parties agree to disclosure.
- Preparation occurs before the exercise begins and includes:
  - definition of roles
  - explicit recognition when players are not being themselves e.g. changing names, gender and change from real life roles
  - predetermination of at least the start of a 'script' or a theme for the discussion.
- All participants should be clear when the role play has started, when it is paused and when it has finished.
- Players should be considerate of their fellows and be aware that strong emotions may be produced. It may be necessary for an observer to halt the play.
- Effective feedback techniques are used, perhaps using a structured format.
- Observations are more helpful than judgements.
- Criticism should be of behaviours not individuals.
- Debriefing of all participants is essential. At the end of the role play a check should be made that all participants are 'back' as themselves and not carrying with them features of the role they had adopted, that any issues arising have been addressed or there is an agreed plan to address them. In trio work, the observer will usually take special responsibility for this.

# References

1    Brookfield SD. *Understanding and Facilitating Adult Learning.* Milton Keynes: Open University Press; 1986.

2    Secretary of State for Health. Trust, Assurance and Safety – the regulation of health professionals in the 21st century. London: The Stationery Office; 2007.

3    Knowles M. *Self-directed Learning.* Cambridge: Adult Education; 1976.

4    Mohanna K, Wall D, Chambers R. *Teaching Made Easy: a manual for health professionals.* 2nd ed. Oxford: Radcliffe Medical Press; 2004.

5   Tuckman B. Original 'Forming-storming-norming-performing' concept; 1965. Summarised by Chapman A, at www.businessballs.com (accessed 3.1.07).

6   Taraschi R. Cutting the Ties that Bind. *Training 101*. Alexandria, Virginia; American Society for Training & Development (ASTD): 2001.

7   Bourner T, Martin V, Race P. Workshops that Work: 100 ideas to make your training events more effective. In: Bennett R, editor. *The McGraw-Hill Training Series*. McGraw-Hill; 2005.

8   Arnold KJ. How to build your expertise in facilitation. In: Schuman S, editor. *The IAF Handbook of Group Facilitation.* San Fransisco: Jossey-Bass; 2005.

Chapter 5

# The official curriculum teacher

*David Wall*

> This teacher is very well prepared as a teacher, is accredited, very aware of and teaches to the formal curriculum and follows external targets for teaching.

Teachers who are comfortable in this style understand the importance of being well prepared as a teacher. They will have planned and prepared the sessions to be taught well in advance, having all the materials there and being familiar with how to use them, their preparation fits in with what is meant to be covered in the curriculum.

The teacher has also been trained to teach, and has attended and completed appropriate 'teaching the teachers' courses (or faculty development). This teacher is very familiar with the formal curriculum statements underpinning the teaching (which may be the aims and objectives of a single course, such as a family planning course, or an advanced life support course, or may be the external curriculum of an institution such as that of a Royal College or faculty, or that of a national body – such as the Modernising Medical Careers initiative and the Foundation Curriculum). All of these may be regarded as external targets in teaching.

As well as being familiar with the curriculum statements, this teacher is very careful to match their teaching with these curriculum statements, so that over the course of time, the whole curriculum has been properly covered. As well as being familiar with the curriculum, such a teacher will have a good understanding of what curriculum is, understands the different models of curriculum, and what is involved in the formal curriculum, the informal curriculum and the hidden curriculum.

## What does this style mean?

This teaching style sets great store by faculty development. We will look at whether teaching the teachers courses work. Do they in fact help teachers to improve their teaching knowledge and skills? What other effects do they have? What should be taught on such courses?

Similarly we will look at aspects of curriculum; what models of curriculum there are and list their strengths and weaknesses. What model should we be using today? Are there any good examples of such curricula? Are there any bad examples of such curricula, so we can see how not to do it? How can we evaluate a curriculum to see if it fits our needs as an official curriculum teacher? These issues are discussed below.

## Do teaching the teachers courses help?

The answer from the medical education literature is 'yes they do'. Box 5.1 shows several examples in the literature illustrating that they do improve teaching, do help teachers enjoy their teaching more, and that teachers become more active in educational planning as well. Learners can detect the differences between those who have been trained to teach and those who have not.

---

**Box 5.1 Some studies to support these views.**

Whitehouse followed up participants who had attended a six day educational *teaching the teachers* course.[1] The follow up showed changes for the better. A group of keen educators resulted from the courses which continues to meet up to the present time, as the Warwickshire Bosworth Group.

In Turkey, Yolsal *et al* reported the impact of their six to nine day *training of trainers* courses since 1997.[2] Medical teachers said that they had implemented the knowledge and skills acquired on the courses, and that students had given better feedback on their teaching. Many stated that they now enjoyed their teaching more, and that they had set up a network of keen teachers as a result of being on the courses together.

Steinert *et al* at McGill University in Canada described a year long faculty development programme to develop leaders in medical education.[3] The course included educational knowledge and skills, in protected time, while maintaining the participants' other clinical, teaching and research responsibilities. A year after completing the programme, the authors found in a follow up survey of 22 faculty members that many had joined new educational committees, taken up new leadership roles in medical education and developed new courses for students and doctors in training. Two had pursued further studies to Masters level.

However, all three studies relied on self reporting by the participants themselves rather than objective evidence.

---

More recent studies used different methodologies and other end point assessments to make similar points. Godfrey, Dennick and Welsh from Sheffield, asked whether a 'teaching the teachers' course did in fact develop teaching skills.[4] They used a quasi-experimental design, and compared a group of medical consultant teachers who underwent a three day teaching the teachers course with a control group taken from the course waiting list. However, participants were not randomly assigned to the taught group or the control group. A questionnaire of teaching skills was applied to participants and controls before the course and at 8–10 months afterwards. Up to 63% of participants and 51% of controls replied to all aspects of this study. Those who had attended the course did significantly better and reported significantly greater improvements in teaching skills. Self reporting was a source of bias, but the control group in this research design did help overcome these issues.

Morrison *et al* in a Californian study, ran a 13 hour teaching the teachers course over six months. [5] The outcome measures included the participants being assessed by trained medical students. A sub-set of the participants were interviewed one year later by two educational researchers, who did not know in advance who had attended the course and who was a control. Those residents in the teaching the teachers course group did significantly better and people who were required to attend did as well as those who volunteered. The interviews showed that the taught group showed greater enthusiasm for teaching one year on, used learner-centred approaches, and had more elaborate understanding of pedagogic principles, and planned to teach after finishing their training.

In Alberta, Pandachuck compared a group of medical teachers who had attended 'teaching the teachers' workshops compared with controls (who had not) by means of ratings by medical students on their teaching abilities before and after the workshops.[6] Students' ratings of teachers' teaching abilities increased significantly for the teachers after the workshops, but remained unchanged for the control group, who had not attended the workshops.

Most recently new evidence from the Best Evidence Medical Education (BEME) review of faculty development initiatives[7] showed that overall satisfaction with programmes was high; participants reported positive changes in attitude to teaching; increased knowledge of educational principles and of gains in teaching skills; changes in teaching behaviours; and greater educational involvement and establishment of collegiate networks. Key strategies for effective interventions to improve teaching effectiveness in medical education included experiential learning; feedback; effective peer and colleague relationships; interventions which followed the principles of teaching and learning; and the use of a wide variety of educational methods.

So, there is now very good evidence from several sources that teaching the teachers courses do work to improve teaching knowledge and skills, can increase teacher enjoyment of teaching, and do produce changes in teacher behaviours for the better.

## What should be taught to teachers to help them be better teachers?

What should be taught on such courses? Two studies using different research designs have given very similar answers (see Box 5.2). Gibson and Campbell carried out a population study on all 869 hospital consultants in Northern Ireland in 2000. [8] Their aim was to help hospital consultants identify their needs in relation to teaching skills. They used a postal questionnaire and focus groups. The researchers concluded from the questionnaire that the main areas that individuals wished to have further training in were: small group work; problem based learning; service based learning; basic teaching skills; and in assessment and appraisal skills. The key themes identified from the focus group were basic teaching skills; appraisal and assessment; giving feedback; small group teaching; and problem orientated learning.

The researchers concluded that there was a hierarchy of need for teaching the teachers training. All consultants needed to have a basic level of instruction, and those with educational jobs such as clinical tutors or Royal College tutors needed more. The most involvement was needed for those who had a major input into medical education, who should therefore need a higher qualification in this area. This was a study of hospital consultants only, but did not involve their learners, i.e. the hospital doctors and dentists in training.

---

**Box 5.2 What should teaching the teachers courses include?**

In 2000, Wall and McAleer reported their work on consultants as teachers. [9]

The study was a mixed methods design, with in-depth interviews of experts, consultants and junior doctors to identify key topics. A literature review and analyses of existing teaching the teachers courses were triangulated to produce a questionnaire. This questionnaire was sent to all senior and junior doctors in four hospitals in the West Midlands Deanery. The top five themes identified as being key to good teaching were:

1 giving feedback constructively
2 keeping up to date as a teacher
3 building a good educational climate
4 assessing the trainees
5 assessing the trainees' learning needs.

This study used different methods but produced similar findings to that of Gibson and Campbell. [8] As well as the consultants, this study took into account the views of the learners themselves, the young doctors in training. However, it is interesting to note that the views of the trainees matched very closely those of the consultants with no significant differences between the two groups.

---

So from both the studies reported in Box 5.2, the themes of giving feedback constructively, assessment and appraisal skills, building a good educational climate, and basic teaching skills using a variety of methods were what teachers and learners wanted to be taught.

Such teachers, well trained in these teaching techniques, should be able to use a variety of teaching methods, and choose and use the most appropriate one for the teaching situation they are operating within. So they would not attempt to teach a practical skill using a lecture based course, or test communication skills with a multiple choice question paper, or do what I have been asked to do on many occasions, to come and give a lecture on communication skills.

## Understanding about curriculum will help

What about curriculum theory? Two commonly held models of the curriculum are the objectives model,[10] and the process model.[11] The objectives model views education as a means to an end. Objectives are set out in advance, and are usually written in behavioural terms, of what the learner is expected to be able to do at the end of the course and training proceeds to instruct the learners in these skills.[12] The model is good for teaching manual skills and tasks within medicine (such as resuscitation skills) where a set of responses in a specified order is used. Such a model of training does not need the doctor to make informed decisions, only to perform a set of responses in a specified order.

However, the objectives model has been criticised because it focuses on knowledge (knowing what) and does not account for nurturing thinking skills and understanding (knowing how). The process model was developed to meet these concerns. Such a model may have greater educational value, since it shifts the learner to the understanding, analysis, synthesis and evaluation of concepts and behaviours as opposed to

> the mere acquisition of predetermined knowledge ... offering a rigid syllabus of content or a fixed hierarchy of objectives to be achieved ...[13]

The role of the teacher becomes more important, since high quality teaching and facilitation focusing on understanding and giving justification for actions taken is essential. There is much to be said for the process model.

More recently there has been much discussion about competences and meta-competences, or outcomes.[14,15,16] Competences differ from behavioural objectives in terms of the much greater broadness of what a competency encompasses, compared to a behavioural objective (see above). A competency has been defined as

> ... a combination of attributes such as knowledge, skills and attitudes underlying some aspect of successful professional performance ...[17]

It also encompasses much more, and involves a person's ability and willingness to get their act together, coordinating their cognitive, affective and other resources in the performance of a professional task.[17]

This outcomes based curriculum movement has built on the process model of the curriculum. Curricula have been written using various outcomes, such as the 'Scottish Doctor' with twelve outcomes,[18] and the CanMEDS 2000 competences, with seven outcomes.[19]

The objectives model works well for technical skills, but is much less useful for process, such as communication, empathy, probity etc. It also has the disadvantage of leading to a large list of objectives as curriculum writers attempt to cover everything. If on the other hand, we look at the CanMEDS competences, as an example of a process or outcomes curriculum, the list is much shorter, is written within one page, and does tackle these other areas well.

Very recently, the new curriculum for general medical practice in the United Kingdom, from the Royal College of General Practitioners, has been published. It defines the core competences to become a general practitioner. It uses an outcomes based model, and describes its learning outcomes in terms of six domains of competence.[20]

Increasing understanding of the curriculum, has led to a move from the early objectives models, through process and now to outcomes based models of curriculum used increasingly in our teaching and learning and in assessment. However, some are still using the objectives model to describe complex behavioural processes. This makes it much more difficult for the individual medical teacher to grasp what is needed when trying to teach according to the official curriculum.

## Is this style really you?

If you like to have the security of knowing that what you are teaching is all prescribed in the curriculum, that you are covering the curriculum in a systematic way, and that what you are teaching about will match the curriculum and the assessments (what is called blueprinting)[17] then this style is for you. It means that you will have a copy of the curriculum to which you refer, that you plan the teaching accordingly, and that you assess the learner along the same lines. This is all helped of course if your teaching documentation follows the same educational concepts in its design. It is much more difficult if it does not.

In terms of curriculum, you will be a strong advocate of the *official* curriculum as a means of systematically covering the curriculum rather than the *informal* curriculum, aspects gathered during activities learners might organise for themselves, such as a journal club. You may not be a supporter of the *hidden* curriculum or aspects learners learn along the way, often by role modelling, which can include the null curriculum – things the institution definitely does not intend to teach – such as rudeness, dishonesty and arrogance.

In deriving the six teaching styles, the group which loaded most strongly onto the official curriculum style in our study were dentists. This may be because the professional development portfolio, used as a record of vocational training in general dental practice in England and Wales, is designed around a small number of key skills, which everyone has been taught on the trainers' courses. The portfolio which the vocational dental practitioners use to record their learning fits very well with this model.

## Making the most of your preferred style

If the official curriculum teacher is your preferred style, then you should ensure that you have been well trained as a teacher. So you will have attended and enjoyed such teaching the teachers courses. You may even have taken this further and have a university qualification in medical education, such as a certificate, diploma or Masters degree in medical education. Most of those doing such courses do them in order to become a better teacher, not to be an education researcher.[21]

You also will need to have studied the curriculum for the courses you are going to teach, and you will be very clear (from reading, from communicating with other colleagues and from feedback from learners) about what you will be teaching and how you will be teaching it, using the best and most appropriate methods to teach those topics in the official curriculum. You will design your lesson plans well in advance, and have all your materials ready before the course takes place, with all handout materials ready at the start of the sessions. You will probably have a bank of teaching materials that you can draw upon in this regard. You will not rely on informal teaching, or expect the learners to catch and capture important concepts along the way, but will ensure that such topics are in your teaching plans, and are taught. Your teaching and learning will fit in not just with the curriculum, but also with the assessments (if the whole course has been designed properly), and if it has not, you will be making strong representations for the three main aspects (curriculum, teaching and learning and assessment) all to 'blueprint' onto each other.

## Improving this style if it is your least preferred style

Curriculum, teaching and learning and assessment should all match, and all 'blueprint' onto each other.[17] Often they do not. Bullock *et al* researched four specialties (accident and emergency medicine, cardiac surgery, ENT surgery and paediatrics) in terms of curriculum, teaching and learning, and assessment.[22] In three of the areas, the curriculum was hardly if ever referred to, teaching and learning was on whatever came through the door and assessments were largely unconnected with both curriculum and teaching and learning.

So, if you want to improve your official curriculum style, using simple concepts, maps and models of education will help you a lot. Use these theoretical frameworks to plan your teaching sessions. This has been known and written about for some years now. As Parry described, a surgeon in training had commented that

> … relating aims, methods and assessment of outcome to be a useful starting point in assessing medical education and noted that most clinical teachers lacked even this degree of structure in their thinking …[23]

Next, obtain the course or curriculum documents and find out what you are supposed to be doing. One way to do this is to use a well established framework to evaluate the course or curriculum, e.g. Harden's ten questions.[24] The simple framework in Figure 5.1 allows you to do this yourself. Try this out on your next course and see if you can write an answer in each of the ten comments boxes.

1 **What are the needs in relation to the product of the training programme?**
Needs of the programme in relation to what is wanted as an end product – fit for purpose – may consult experts, errors in practice, critical incident reports, task analysis, morbidity and mortality figures, opinions and beliefs of star performers, looking at existing curricula and views of recent students.

2 **What are the aims and objectives?**
What are the overall aims, and in more detail the objectives as to what the person will be able to do at the end of the course of study

3 **What content should be included?**
Content gets put in if:

- it directly contributes to the course objectives
- it is a building block of skill or knowledge needed to tackle a later part of the course
- it allows development of intellectual abilities such as critical thinking
- it aids the understanding of other subjects on the course.

4 **How should the content be organised?**
This relates to the order in which subjects are taught – and a theoretical plan of why the order is organised as it is.

5 **What educational strategies should be adopted?**
These relate to the model of curriculum being used, such as in medical education the SPICES model,[25] the spiral curriculum, an objectives model, a process model and an outcome based model. Sometimes there is no obvious model at all!

6 **What teaching methods should be adopted?**
Student grouping may be one way, with for example, either whole class teaching by the lecture method, small groups, one to one bedside teaching, distance learning and so on. Another way may be by teaching and learning tools, such as computer packages, web based learning, simulators, skills laboratories role-play and so on. Obviously the choices of methods need to reflect the course aims and objectives and so on. One would not choose to teach communication skills and breaking bad news to patients in a lecture-based course.

7 **How should assessment be carried out?**
These include the choice of assessments used (such as essays, projects, portfolios, MCQs, OSCEs, oral examinations, long and short cases and so on. Who will assess the work? Are there external examiners? Is there self-assessment? Will assessment be continuous through-out the course or at the end? What are the standards to be achieved? Are the assessment standards criterion referenced or norm referenced? Finally how is the course evaluated? Is it by the students? Is there internal and external evaluation?

8 **How should details of the curriculum be communicated?**
Details have to be communicated to those teaching the course, the students attending the course, potential students and other bodies. How is this done? How do the subjects relate to each other and the final product?

9 **What educational environment or climate should be fostered?**
Does the environment encourage cooperation between students, students and teachers, scholarship, probity and support, or is it hostile, with teaching by humiliation, sexism and bullying?

10 **How should the process be managed?**
Who is responsible for planning, organising and managing the process? Can changes be made? How does this course relate to others? Is there student representation? Do the teaching staff know what is going on? Is there a course committee?

Assessment sheet using Harden's ten questions for the analysis of the curriculum statements for university educational courses.

| | |
|---|---|
| 1 What are the needs in relation to the product of the training programme? | |
| 2 What are the aims and objectives? | |
| 3 What content is included? | |
| 4 How is the content organised? | |
| 5 What educational strategies are adopted? | |
| 6 What teaching methods are adopted? | |
| 7 How is assessment carried out? | |
| 8 How are details of the curriculum communicated? | |
| 9 What educational environment or climate is fostered? | |
| 10 How is the process managed? | |

**Figure 5.1** Ten questions to ask when planning a course or curriculum. (Adapted by David Wall from: Harden RM. Ten questions to ask when planning a course or curriculum. *Med Educ.* 1986; **20**: 356–65.)

Then, plan the course according to the above, making sure that you cover what is there. Take account of the best ways to teach such things, which you should have learned about on your teaching the teachers courses, and ask colleagues about this as well. Have all your plans and materials ready, before the course takes place. If you are going to teach on a particular topic, then have it all prepared, and do not rely on suitable patients turning up in the ward, the clinic or the surgery as if by magic just as you begin to teach. All of this needs organisation well beforehand.

On the course itself, adhere to your plans, stick to your timetable, and do what you intended to do. Do not get sidetracked into irrelevant issues, no matter how interesting these may be. Think carefully about the subject to be taught and the best way to facilitate this. If your main preferred style is that of a sensitive student-centred teacher, then resist the temptation to teach everything sitting in circles in small groups using drama and role play. This is not the best way to teach a practical skill.

Once the course has taken place, evaluate the course by learners' opinions and by yourself (self evaluation), giving your own honest reflections on what went well, what went not so well and why, and write down ideas for improvements next time. Feed these into the design that you did at the beginning. Hopefully all this will help you strengthen your official curriculum teaching style.

# References

1   Whitehouse A. Warwickshire consultants' 'training the trainers' course. *Postgrad Med*. 1997; **73**: 35–8.

2   Yolsal N, Bulut A, Karabey S, *et al*. Development of training of trainers programmes and evaluation of their effectiveness in Istanbul, Turkey. *Med Teach*. 2003; **25**: 319–24.

3   Steinert Y, Nasmith L, McLeod PJ, *et al*. A teaching scholars program to develop leaders in medical education. *Acad Med*. 2003; **78**: 142–9.

4   Godfrey J, Dennick R, Welsh, C. Training the trainers: do teaching courses develop teaching skills? *Med Educ*. 2004; **38**: 844–7.

5   Morrison EH, Rucker L, Boker JR, *et al*. The effect of a 13 hour curriculum to improve residents' teaching skills: a randomized trial. *Ann Intern Med*. 2004; **141**: 257–63.

6   Pandachuck K, Harley D, Cook D. Effectiveness of a brief workshop designed to improve teaching performance at the University of Alberta. *Acad Med*. 2004; **79**: 798–804.

7   Steinert Y, Mann K, Centeno A, *et al*. A systematic review of faculty development initiatives designed to improve teaching effectiveness in medical education: BEME Guide No. 8. *Med Teach*. 2006; **28**: 497–526.

8   Gibson DR, Campbell RM. Promoting effective teaching and learning: hospital consultants identify their needs. *Med Educ*. 2000; **34**: 126–30.

9   Wall D, McAleer S. Teaching the consultant teachers: identifying the core content. *Med Educ*. 2000; **34**: 131–8.

10 Rowntree D. *Educational technology in Curriculum Development*. 2nd ed. London: Paul Chapman Publishing; 1982.

11 Stenhouse N. *An Introduction to Curriculum Research and Development*. Oxford: Heinemann Educational Publications; 1975.

12 Mohanna K, Wall D, Chambers R. *Teaching Made Easy: a manual for health professionals*. 2nd ed. Oxford: Radcliffe Medical Press; 2004.

13 Kelly AV. The *Curriculum Theory and Practice*. 3rd ed. London; Paul Chapman Publishing; 1989.

14 Ross N, Davies D. Outcomes based learning and the electronic curriculum. *Med Teach*. 1999; **21**: 23–5.

15 Harden RM, Crosby JR, Davis MH. An introduction to outcomes based education. *Med Teach*. 1999; **21**: 7–14.

16 Harden RM, Crosby JR, Davis MH, *et al*. From competency to meta-competency – a model for the specification of learning outcomes. *Med Teach*. 1999; **21**: 546–52.

17 Dent JA, Harden RM. *A Practical Guide for Medical Teachers*. 2nd ed. Edinburgh: Elsevier Churchill Livingstone; 2005.

18 Simpson JG, Furnace J, Crosby J, *et al*. The Scottish Doctor – learning outcomes for the medical undergraduate in Scotland: a foundation for competent and reflective practitioners. *Med Teach*. 2002; **2**: 136–43.

19 CanMEDS. CanMEDS 2000 Project. Skills for the New Millennium Report of the Societal Needs Working Group. Royal College of Physicians and Surgeons of Canada. Ottawa, Ontario, Canada Heinemann Educational Publications. 1996.

20 Royal College of General Practitioners. *GP Curriculum Documents*. London: Royal College of General Practitioners. 2006. http://www.rcgp.org.uk/education_/education_home/curriculum/gp_curriculum_documents.aspx (accessed 24th Jan 2007).

21 Allery L, Brigley S, MacDonald J, *et al*. *Degrees of Difference: An investigation of Masters and Doctorate Programmes in Medical Education*. Edinburgh: Association for the Study of Medical Education; 2005.

22 Bullock A, Burke S, Wall D. Curriculum and assessment in higher specialist training. *Med Teach*. 2004; **26**: 174–7.

23 Parry KM. The doctor as teacher. *Med Educ*. 1987; **21**: 512–20.

24 Harden RM. Approaches to curriculum planning. *Med Educ*. 1986; **20**: 458–66.

25 Harden R, Sowden S, Dunn WR. *Some educational strategies in curriculum development: the SPICES model*. ASME medical educational booklet 18. Dundee: Centre for Medical Education; 1984.

# Chapter 6

# The straight facts no nonsense teacher

*David Wall*

> This teacher likes to teach the clear facts, with straight talking, concentrating on specific skills, and much prefers not to be involved with multiprofessional teaching and learning.

So this style is about the person who enjoys their teaching, who likes to teach the clear facts, in simple language, which is often very popular with people who are just beginning the subject, the novices at both undergraduate and postgraduate level. Here, the clear facts as a basic framework are useful for the learners to establish a framework on which to place other more complex concepts.

## What does this style mean?

This teacher has often distilled the subject to be taught into a small number of key principles, the basic maps and models of the subject as a foundation to the subject. This is delivered with straight talking, applied to these key points. This teacher also loves to teach specific skills, and has thought a lot about the teaching of such skills, again often having distilled the skill down to a series of small steps, which they will then impart to the learner (see Box 6.1).

Such a teacher will be most happy teaching young learners in their profession the 'right' way to do things. They will be less happy in a multi-disciplinary setting, teaching and interacting with other professions within the health service or teaching lay people about medical matters.

Basic knowledge and skills are very important. They are the foundations on which the rest of healthcare practice is based. Without these strong foundations, there is little hope of building the higher level functioning required for practice.

Some may think that this teaching style and this concept is now outdated, particularly for postgraduate training. Some may say that healthcare students entering practice-based training grades should know the basic facts, and that we should aim to teach at a higher level of competence or performance. However, as one example of how this is not always the case, a recent study of newly qualified doctors showed that they felt well prepared in communication skills, but much less prepared in decision making, diagnosis,

---

**Box 6.1 Contrasting teaching styles – a personal example.**

As a medical student, many years ago now, David can vividly remember such teachers, who were very popular with the students.

'From such teachers we learned our basic clinical knowledge and skills, being taught usually a single way to do things, as the one correct way to do it. People who did things differently were criticised, and could be failed in examinations for using the wrong technique. It was thus a great surprise and shock to me, as a final year medical student on my elective in southern Africa, seeing other students and doctors doing these skills equally well if not better, having been taught them in a different way and using different techniques.

'For example, I had always been taught that to perform a lumbar puncture or an epidural injection, the patient must be curled up on a bed in the left lateral position. I was very surprised to see this expertly done with the patient sitting the "wrong way round" on a chair, using the back of the chair to support the patient leaning forwards, with their arms folded and resting on the back of the chair. This method worked extremely well, especially for women in labour. This was a seminal moment for me, realising for the first time that there were probably many correct methods and ways to do things in medicine, not just one, and that this concept could be applied to many situations.'

---

prescribing and other basic doctoring skills.[1] This finding was confirmed by their consultant educational supervisors. In fact one commented that

> … I feel we train good communicators who often lack the base knowledge of what they need to communicate.

The teacher competent in this teaching style may be most comfortable with a model of teaching that is content-based. This teacher excels in explaining the building blocks of future knowledge, mastery of which (application, flexibility, adaptability) might come at a later stage.

The importance of a step-wise progression of learning is recognised in two educational models, Bloom's Taxonomy of the knowledge domain,[2] and Miller's pyramid.[3] Both of these are described in Box 6.2.

In 1956, Bloom and a team of educationalists described a classification of learning, in three domains, a *cognitive* domain, a *psychomotor* domain, and an *affective* domain, which may more simply be expressed as knowledge, skills and attitudes.[4] The cognitive domain (knowledge) is expressed as a six step hierarchy, as shown in Figure 6.1. Note that knowledge forms the base, and successive levels of learning build on this base.

In terms of a psychomotor domain, of skills, Bloom did not produce a taxonomy for this area of learning. Others have since done so.[5,6,7] However we can use a model which has a similar hierarchy that can be used to classify skills

---

**Box 6.2 Step-wise learning.**

**Teaching the facts – in a knowledge domain.**

Teaching basic facts in isolation can make learning harder than it needs to be. Bloom's Taxonomy reminds us that there is a hierarchy of learning within each of the three domains of learning. For example, let us take the concept of atrial fibrillation. You can teach knowledge about it at a basic level. But you can also extend learners to be able to analyse that information, by asking what happens as a result of atrial fibrillation. Still further levels of sophistication are required to apply that learning if we ask how it is treated to prevent some of the complications. There are many studies in this area, of anticoagulation and prevention of stroke and other embolic events, and the synthesis and evaluation of these have brought us up to the highest levels in Bloom's Taxonomy in the cognitive (knowledge) domain. If the learners can see the relevance in learning about the basic facts, by applying them, then they may remember these facts in context better than as isolated things to remember for the exam and be forgotten afterwards.

**Teaching the facts – in a skills domain.**

Similarly in terms of skills, the hierarchy of the Miller's pyramid may be utilised by the straight facts no nonsense teacher. In learning a particular skill, performing a hysterectomy perhaps, the learner can be taken through the steps of knowing the anatomy of the pelvis and what a hysterectomy is (knows), then seeing it done and assisting, knowing what the basic steps are, and the pitfalls to avoid (knows how), then doing it with a lot of help (shows how), and then being able to perform the operation in a capable way (does). Again, the basic facts are very important, knowing the anatomy, having the basic surgical skills of dissection, use of instruments, tying knots securely and so on, before you can take the learner through to the next levels, to eventually become an expert performer in that area. This teaching style is excellent for moving learners up towards higher levels of learning by ensuring the basics are in place.

---

in terms of basic knowledge through to mastery, called Miller's pyramid.[8] This is illustrated in Figure 6.2. In many situations, in particular with regard to assessment in education, this model is used to assess skills. Again, note that, as in Bloom's Taxonomy above, the base, the foundation of the model is knowledge (knows). Next is the application of knowledge (knows how), then competence (shows how) and at the top, performance (does).

Although Miller described the model, with four levels, Dent and Harden added a fifth level, at the top of the pyramid, which they called *mastery*, to denote the difference between being able to perform a skill, and being able to perform that skill in an expert and masterful way.[3]

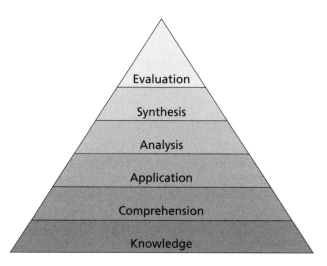

**Figure 6.1** Bloom's Taxonomy model for the cognitive (knowledge) domain.

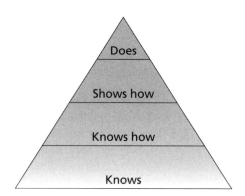

**Figure 6.2** Miller's pyramid of a skills taxonomy.

## Is this style really you?

If you like to teach the clear facts, and are a clear thinker who has thought a lot about your subject and managed to distil it down to a series of simple concepts and step by step actions then this is probably the preferred style for you. You will be a teacher who has thought a lot about the areas that you like to teach, and you will be very clear about the right and wrong answers to questions in these areas. You will like to teach the facts, in the knowledge domain, and specific skills and practical procedures, in the psychomotor domain. You will like to teach in your own specialty, and feel uncomfortable working outside of it. You will like to teach in such areas as advanced life support courses, surgical skills courses and other practical skills based areas. You will probably be highly valued and respected as a skills teacher, within your professional area. At home you might be a very practical person, who would not dream of calling in a plumber to put in a new washbasin or toilet, having all the tools and skills to do this yourself to a high standard.

You will probably be quite uneasy working and teaching in the attitudes domain. You will therefore not be very interested in teaching about the attitudinal aspects of medicine, including communication skills, breaking bad news and so on, or in the specialties where feelings and empathy are to the fore. If you are teaching about such areas as bereavement, or breaking bad news, then again you will have distilled this down into a series of steps, which will be done in a mechanistic way, with not a lot of regard for what the patient, the relatives or the nurses are feeling about the situation. Of course, you would much prefer to leave such areas to be handled and taught by the communications skills people, the nurses, midwives and general practitioners.

# Making the most of this as your preferred style

If the clear facts no nonsense teacher is your preferred style, then there are various concepts, maps and models and techniques that will help you to be even better in your preferred style.

In terms of teaching a practical skill, then the *set, dialogue* and *closure* method is a useful one which allows you to break the skill down and to teach it in a series of small steps.[2] The teaching of a practical skill can be looked on as both imparting a new skill to a learner and also for a discussion about the topic in general terms. Time is often limited and therefore it is essential that an adequate knowledge base has been covered in advance.

The three basic steps are as follows:

1 set: the preparation stage
2 dialogue: the procedure itself
3 closure: the reflection, critique, feedback, and planning the next steps for the next session.

### The three steps in detail

Set: preparation

This is a very important part of the whole process. It is essential to think of and define precise objectives for the session. How does the skill being taught here identify with other learning events which have been taught recently? You as the teacher must decide what form the teaching will take, and plan the environment meticulously. This will include the location, the lighting, the seating position and all the equipment you will use for the teaching session. You must ensure that the learner is familiar with the arrangements and knows what you are going to do beforehand. So, if you are going to teach about a surgical procedure, make sure that the learner knows about this in advance, and has had the opportunity to read up on the procedure beforehand.

Dialogue: the procedure

The method is a four step model of talking through and demonstrating the practical skill. It is divided into four steps. These are as follows:

1 teacher performs the task without commentary, at a normal speed
2 teacher performs the procedure again, slowly, talking the way through it
3 learner talks the procedure through, while teacher does it again
4 learner talks through the procedure while the learner does it.

Obviously this is the sort of procedure that could take place in a skills lab using models, rather than with a real patient having the procedure done four times! However, adaptations of this four step model can be used in real life, with real patients. You can talk the procedure through before carrying it out, talking your way through it with the learner, and then getting the learner to talk it through, before doing it.

Closure: the summary

After the procedure has been successfully carried out, then this is the opportunity to reflect on the procedure, give feedback, tips, ask and answer questions and plan what you are going to do next time. Here is a very good opportunity to give the learner some tricks of the trade, the little tips which can make all the difference between success and failure of a procedure. These may be things you have learned the hard away, over many years, which you can hand on to the next generation.

## Learning this method of teaching a practical skill

A useful and enjoyable method of learning this structured method of teaching is to practise teaching a practical skill with your colleagues using microteaching sessions. Ask the learners to bring the props to teach a simple non-work related skill to one of their colleagues, which can be taught in a five minute microteaching session. Use the set, dialogue and closure method.

Over the years I have observed many such sessions, including how to put on a turban, how to make a trifle, paper folding, fly tying, knot tying, tree pruning, how to make Irish coffee, and how to develop a good golf swing. All of these have been great fun, and have worked well. One tip, however, is to watch the lights in the ceiling when swinging the golf club, especially in a room with a low ceiling! We know about this from bitter experience.

## Giving feedback constructively

In these teaching situations above, there is the need to be able to give feedback to the learner. A useful method of giving feedback constructively in such situations in busy clinical work is to use the method known as the *one minute teacher* (called the *one minute preceptor* in the USA – but in the United Kingdom *teacher* is much more commonly used and understood). [9]

The model is in five steps, which the authors called 'five microskills for clinical teaching,' as follows:

1  **get a commitment**. Ask, 'what do you think is going on here?'
   Asking the learner how they interpreted the situation you are teaching
   them about in the work place is the first step in diagnosing their learning
   needs

2  **probe for supporting evidence**. Ask, 'what led you to that conclusion?'
   Ask the learner for their evidence before offering your opinion. Probe their
   current knowledge and skills. This will allow you to find out about what
   they know and identify where they have gaps

3  **teach general rules and principles**. 'When this happens, do this...'
   Instruction will be remembered better if in the form of a general rule or
   principle

4  **reinforce what was right and be specific**. 'You did an excellent job of...'
   Reinforce their knowledge and skills especially when these are not well
   established and give praise as appropriate to motivate them

5  **correct mistakes**. 'Next time this happens try this instead ...'
   Mistakes that are left unattended have a good chance of being repeated.

Bedside teaching, teaching in the clinic and outpatients department and in
the operating theatre are all in busy clinical environments. This method of
giving constructive feedback quickly is very useful in such situations, is much
quicker than the Pendleton's Rules model of giving feedback constructively,[10]
and is well worth trying out. It does really work!

## Improving this style if it is your least preferred style

If this is your least preferred style, then you are probably happier teaching in
other ways such as through small groups, using role play and in-depth discussions about emotions and feelings, or in the opposite way, giving a didactic
lecture.

So, if you want to improve your straight facts no nonsense style, in your
knowledge and skills teaching, stick to your plans, stick to your techniques,
and do what you intended to do. Do not get sidetracked into other issues, no
matter how interesting these may be to you. If your main preferred style is
that of a sensitive student-centred teacher, then resist the temptation to teach
everything sitting in circles in small groups using drama and role play. This is
not the best way to teach basic knowledge and practical skills. Neither is the
didactic lecture, much favoured by the big conference teacher, the best way
to teach someone how to do a hysterectomy.

Once your teaching has taken place, evaluate the teaching yourself by
reflecting on your own honest observations on what went well, what went
not so well and why, and write down ideas for improvements next time.
Enhance this by asking for learners' opinions. Feed these in to the lesson plan
that you did at the beginning.

You could also consider enrolling yourself in teaching the teachers training,
to work at understanding the concepts which are being taught there, and to

use them in your teaching. In particular, pay attention to Bloom's Taxonomy and Miler's pyramid.

Make sure that you take part in microteaching or observation of teaching sessions, particularly on how to teach a practical skill perhaps using the set, dialogue and closure method described above.

Using these simple concepts, and maps and models of education, will help you a lot. Using these theoretical frameworks to plan your teaching sessions, and plan what you are going to do, will enhance your performance in this teaching style.

# References

1  Wall D, Bolshaw A, Carolan J. From undergraduate medical education to pre-registration house officer year: how prepared are students? *Med Teach.* 2006; **28**: 435–9.

2  Mohanna K, Wall D, Chambers R. *Teaching Made Easy*: a manual for health professionals. 2nd ed. Oxford: Radcliffe Medical Press; 2004.

3  Dent JA, Harden RM. *A Practical Guide for Medical Teachers*. 2nd ed. Edinburgh: Elsevier Churchill Livingstone; 2005.

4  Bloom BS, editor. *Taxonomy of educational objectives: the classification of educational goals: Handbook I, cognitive domain*. New York: David McKay; 1956.

5  Simpson EJ. *The Classification of Educational Objectives in the Psychomotor Domain*. Washington, DC: Gryphon House; 1973.

6  Dave RH. Psychomotor Levels. In: Armstrong RJ, editor. *Developing and Writing Behavioral Objectives*. Tucson, Arizona: Educational Innovators Press; 1970.

7  Harrow AJ. *A Taxonomy of the Psychomotor Domain*. New York: David McKay; 1972.

8  Miller GE. The assessment of clinical skills/competence/performance. *Acad Med.* 1990; **65**: S63–7 (supplement article).

9  Gordon K, Meyer B, Irby D. *The One Minute Preceptor: five microskills for clinical teaching*. Seattle: University of Washington; 1996.

10  Pendleton D, Schofield T, Tate P, *et al. The Consultation: an approach to learning and teaching*. Oxford: Oxford Medical Publications; 1984.

# Chapter 7

# The big conference teacher

*Ruth Chambers*

> This teacher likes nothing better than to stand up in front of a big audience and does not like sitting in groups or one to one teaching

Conferences seem to be splendid events when you're new to them. Big conferences are usually pretty costly affairs to attend. Unless they are of the special interest variety or charitably based, the delegate fee of national or international conferences can be several hundreds of pounds/euros/dollars per day. When you take travel and accommodation costs and incidental expenses into account as well as opportunity costs for the piles of work you could be processing instead – you wonder how so many people can afford to attend as many conferences as they do. The trick to rendering them affordable is to get more benefits out of attending than costs. Another way is to minimise the expense – a great way to do that is for you to be invited as a keynote speaker with the conference fee, travel and accommodation expenses paid by the conference organiser.

The benefits might be to do with increasing your prestige if you are presenting at the conference or running a workshop there; or displaying a poster of your work. Your updated CV will include brief details of your conference contribution; the delegates' conference pack will include an abstract of your presentation or workshop (or both?) (and maybe your biography if you are a key name) in the conference programme booklet. The conference will be an opportunity for your personal development and to teach those listening to your presentation or participating in your workshop.

Even if you only have a poster accepted at the conference, there may be an opportunity to teach other delegates. Some big conferences organise poster sessions whereby the poster author(s) stand by their display and in five or so minutes relay the key messages of their work. They can also talk to others informally at the designated poster viewing sessions. This is all part of the general networking you might undertake at the conference.

## What does this style mean?

Big conference teaching means enjoying everyone's attention (or at least tolerating it), leading, inspiring, conveying your vision and views, engaging others in a confident manner, convincing others of your expertise and potential.

## Giving a presentation

If you are the keynote speaker, invited by the conference organiser your purpose may be to draw paying delegates to the conference because of your high profile or prestige. Or, you may be the expert on a topic (or others may consider that you are) and are relaying your new or learned perspectives. It could be that the conference organiser is saving money and the conference lecture format saves paying for additional numbers of break-out rooms, speakers or facilitators.

You know it is your opportunity to impress people and convince them of your message. You could be an inspirational teacher. Giving a big conference lecture may be a way for you to reach out to many people at once, your name in highlights as a backdrop. Who wouldn't listen to what you have to say in these circumstances?

You might have an extrovert personality or enjoy showing off your expertise. It might feed your ego to have hundreds or more people gazing at you as the 'teacher' and finding you interesting. It might nourish your confidence and sense of importance if your keynote status is one of the draws to the conference itself. But the person giving the presentation at a big conference that is packed with hundreds or maybe thousands in the audience, has no choice about the format. The 'big conference' setting implies that the format of the delivery of the teaching is in the control of the organisers who are prescriptive in how they arrange the day – typically starting with a keynote presentation or two, moving on to workshops that may be interspersed with more lectures or presentations. So if you are an introverted type of person, shy and timid you will have to learn to cope in the big conference setting if you want the prestige and opportunities that brings – the chance to influence and get your views and findings heard, and promote your hard work.

## Running a workshop

Teaching via a workshop format is covered in Chapter 8. You have less control at a big conference over the numbers attending your workshop as you are not part of the organisation of the event. If you are a popular speaker, delegates who failed to get a place in your workshop might just barge in and you will have to cope unless there is a way for you to bar the extras – sympathise with Ruth's and Kay's experience as described in Box 7.1.

## Networking

You need many of the same positively confident characteristics of the keynote speaker for successful networking. You must engage others, convince them to view you as an expert and respect your contribution. Your teaching will be indirect compared to the delivery of your presentation, but you will be seizing opportunities to tell others about what you do and your potential usefulness to them.

---

**Box 7.1 A worst case scenario of a 'big conference' workshop.**

Ruth and Kay attended a medical careers conference where they were running two workshops. One of the workshops focused on making a career in general practice. They had proposed a limit of 30 delegates to the conference organiser as they wanted to run it in an interactive format. On the day about 150 delegates squeezed into the room – occupying the 60 chairs, sitting in the aisles, in front of the rows of chairs, standing round the walls etc. No one from security was around to help Ruth and Kay control the numbers of participants – and they just had to get on with the workshop. After a quick chat where they decided to make the best of it, they continued with their brief introductory talks. Then they ran the exercises as a VERY large group activity, getting participants to work in pairs with their neighbours, sharing the handouts one between four. Ruth and Kay facilitated contributions from individuals in the plenary group – sharing their lapel microphone between those speaking from the audience and themselves as facilitators.

## Is this style really you?

If your knees quake just at the thought of standing up and speaking in front of a room full of people, let alone going through the reality of it, then the big conference teaching style is not really your preferred way. But it is possible to overcome your fear, and even harness that rush of adrenaline so that it improves your performance.

---

**Box 7.2 Feel the fear and deliver it anyway.**

One of Ruth's first big presentations was to several thousand delegates at an international conference for family doctors, held in Hong Kong. It was perhaps the second time she had given a talk at any conference, and she was the third keynote speaker that day – addressing the topic of excessive stress on doctors. She had been invited because of the articles she had published in the field, since taking up research into stress a few years before. As she sat on the stage facing the audience awaiting her turn with other keynote speakers, she took in the size of the audience for the first time – fear stirred up her intestines so much that she had to leave the stage abruptly to ease herself before returning to give her presentation. She forced herself into positive thinking, visualised her successful delivery. That fear and positive approach did galvanise her into giving one of the best presentations she had ever done then or since.

Quite often when a charismatic speaker has given a rousing lecture, you can think afterwards 'well what did they actually say?' and not be able to voice a single take home message. If you are not naturally charismatic, you will have to find different ways of holding a large audience's attention – developing your unique selling points. Try narratives relaying personal experiences that touch a chord; or varying your tempo to include unexpected components in your talk, or integrating audiovisual aids that grab people's attention. But the harder that you have to try to hold an audience's attention or make an impact, the less likely it is that being a 'big conference' teacher is your chosen personal teaching style.

Many people are frightened of giving a presentation or speaking in public. Every health professional or manager has to speak to groups of other people at sometime – whether it is during a ward round, or at a multidisciplinary case review or in presenting an interesting case at a postgraduate centre. If you want to be a teacher or disseminate the results of a project, or lead and motivate others – you need to conquer this fear.

Good preparation should remove some of the fear. Think positively and prepare beforehand by imagining yourself giving the speech and everything going well. Try to exude an air of enthusiasm and confidence about the subject of your presentation.

Similarly if the 'big conference' setting is not your preference you may have difficulties forcing yourself to network with others if you are shy and reserved. Even if you know other people you may not feel comfortable making the first contact or renewing your relationship, trying to get their attention riveted on you and your conversation. When you walk through the door to the conference hall and see people milling about, you may want to run away, but force yourself onwards thinking of the expense of getting you so far and the opportunities you will forgo if you are not there to take advantage of them.

## Making the most of this if it is your preferred style

Your big conference style will go a long way to gaining you the prestige and respect you want as an expert in your field if it looks natural. Your charisma will gain you new friends and fans without having to make as much effort as the kind of teacher who has to work hard to gain people's attention, or convey their views convincingly.

If you relay your belief in your messages and passion for your subject, then it should be easier for you to make an impact on others in your audience or networks – to get them to listen to you and consider how what they are hearing applies to them. You are starting to teach them – all you need then is to catalyse them to apply that knowledge or change their behaviour. Look at some of the characteristics of an inspiring teacher in Box 7.3 and consider how they apply to you, or could do so with a bit more practise and thought.

Obtain and keep a list of the names of delegates at a conference – and write in their contact details as you network with them and meet them to talk to. There may be enough enthusiasts who share your interest to create a post-conference network of people working in or developing your specialty area.

---

**Box 7.3 Characteristics of an inspiring teacher.**
(Derived from workshop at leadership skills course run by the
Association for the Study of Medical Education (ASME), 2006)

- exhibit a passionate commitment to values and vision
- enable the learner to perceive the vision and how that relates positively to them
- consistent message
- optimistic and/or positive projection of vision or teaching
- communicate well
- instil trust and respect in learners
- use words that cross cultures
- mastery of their expert area
- energise those listening.

---

You could be the one who starts up such a network – then you'll be at the centre of developments. You might keep in touch through an electronic forum with bulletin boards, video conferencing, a series of telephone conferences that are chaired with a semi-structured agenda etc., or follow-on workshops. You might have a practical output from your networking such as a conference report or book on your field of shared interest.

If there is someone you want to meet, see if someone who knows you both can introduce you. Or join their group and wait until there is a gap in the conversation before asking a question. Concentrate on building rapport, being warm and friendly.[1]

Good networkers:[2]

- put themselves out personally in order to build links
- take the initiative
- make the most of opportunities
- present themselves well
- interest other people in their views or work or fields of expertise
- are genuinely interested in others and their work
- seem comfortable and at ease in different settings
- appear competent in varied circumstances
- will take risks and tolerate rejection from others
- prioritise networking in their everyday lives
- understand systems and organisations and can generalise from one to another
- keep details of their contacts in an organised way.

## Improving this if it is not your preferred style

The effectiveness of any speech or presentation will depend to a large extent on how much effort you put into preparing it. You will improve over time from practice and experience and be less likely to fall into the traps summarised in Box 7.4. Be sure about the exact purpose of the presentation. Jot down your initial ideas in rough and add to them over time. Then organise them into a logical sequence and group your ideas under headings. Expand each of the headings in a way that will suit the target audience. Exude an air of enthusiasm and confidence about the subject.

---

**Box 7.4 What to avoid when new to big conference teaching.**

Don't:
- be too dependent on audio-visual aids and panic when they don't work
- be ill prepared to answer questions and look stupidly ignorant
- put up with poor lighting, being either too dark so that the audience falls asleep or too bright so that slides are difficult to read
- pitch your presentation at the wrong level for the audience, either assuming too much prior knowledge and understanding, or seeming patronisingly simple
- deliver a disjointed presentation without a logical flow through from beginning to end
- look down and avoid eye contact or continually turn your back to the audience whilst gazing at the slides showing on the screen
- read flatly from your notes rather than looking round at the audience whilst speaking in an engaging way
- rock backwards and forwards in your anxiety when speaking into a static microphone at a conference or your voice level will ebb and flow
- run over your allotted time, especially when there are several speakers following on.

---

Start by grabbing the interest of the audience, maintaining their attention and finishing with a memorable ending. Do not open by apologising for your lack of knowledge or for being there or keeping them from food, drink, or freedom.
   Some opening gambits are:

- asking a rhetorical question
- repeating a quote or well known saying
- reciting an anecdote
- telling a joke
- shocking your audience with an unexpected statement or a challenging remark
- making an emphatic statement or providing some facts.

Wear comfortable clothes that you feel will stand up to the audience's scrutiny – you will feel increasingly uncomfortable if you think your clothes are too tight, too short or your underwear can be seen.

Some people write out and read their speeches in full whilst others prefer to be more informal, prompted by notes prepared on cards with key headings. Fix your notes together with a treasury tag if they are on different cards or pages so that you don't mix them up in your anxiety of speaking. Then if you do drop your notes they remain in order together. If you need to read the full text of the speech on the occasion then make the size of the words big enough to be easily readable and highlight key points. Try to avoid simply reading out your presentation and aim to talk simply **to** the audience and not **at** the audience.

Practise your talk beforehand. Time it carefully and make sure you leave enough time to dwell on the main points of interpretation and learning compared to the setting of the scene. Consider recording your practice talk and asking colleagues to comment on it constructively. Take off your watch and place it in a prominent position to remind you to keep to time – do not overrun or there will not be enough time for questions. Try and raise your eyes to scan around the audience whenever you can remember. Fix on one or two people when you are talking. Look up at the back rows to include them in your delivery or those sitting there will feel disconnected from listening to the lecture.

Make sure that you deliver your speech so that your words are distinct. Try not to speak too quickly – even experienced speakers can fall into this trap. Vary your tone and pitch to maintain interest. Your voice must be able to be heard by the people at the back of the audience. Change the pace of your presentation to add interest and variety to your talk. You might try for a dramatic effect by saying nothing and pausing for a while.

Link your talk into previous presentations by arriving early enough to hear them or arranging for a private briefing from the conference organiser before you speak to update you on the presentations and discussions that have gone before.

Write yourself big notices saying 'slow down' if you tend to speak too fast; put timings in big letters in your lecture notes if you tend to deliver your presentation more slowly than planned.

Summarise your main messages. Finish with a well polished relevant conclusion; it might be the answer to the rhetorical question posed at the beginning, the end of a story half told earlier in the presentation, a challenge or action plan for the future; don't just tail off and stop abruptly.

The features you adopt to improve your technique and teaching style when giving conference presentations, apply to networking too. The more convincing you are as an expert in your field, the more you look and sound the part so that they trust in your expertise and potential. The better your timing, then the more effective you will be at networking too.

# References

1   Stone C. *The Ultimate Guide to Successful Networking*. London: Vermilion; 2004.

2   Kenway J, Epstein D, Boden R. *Building Networks*. London: Sage; 2005.

# Chapter 8

# The one-off teacher

*Ruth Chambers*

This teacher likes to deliver small self-contained bits of teaching, on a
one to one basis, with no props to help and no follow up

A teacher with a one-off teaching style will take advantage of any formal or
informal opportunity to teach others on a one-off basis. This type of teacher
likes to deliver one-off self-contained topics or sessions without follow up of
the learners. One-off teaching includes giving a lecture to a few or many
people; running a workshop on a one-off basis maybe as a teacher parachuted
in to a group of learners whom they have not met before, nor will meet again;
or any impromptu teaching episode that is not part of a planned series of
learning activities.

## One-off teaching

### The lecture

The advantages of a lecture are well established. A lecture format allows one
expert to share his or her expertise with a great many learners in a short time;
it is relatively cheap in terms of resources – one room and one expert serve
many learners. The syllabus of a course can be covered quickly with a series
of lectures by the same person or a sequence of experts; the lecturer can cover
a lot of ground or clarify difficult concepts. A lecture is a good choice of
format when the topic is new and little has been written about the subject.
The lecturer's enthusiasm for the topic may be infectious and motivate learners to find out more.

But there are many disadvantages to a lecture format too: the audience sits
passively listening to the speaker and may typically lose their concentration
after ten minutes or so. There may be no or little opportunity to ask
questions; many learners' natural reticence prevents them from asking
questions in front of others in case they look stupid. The lecturer goes at the
same pace for all learners and so may deliver the presentation too fast or too
slowly for individuals in the audience and the talk is unlikely to be at the right
depth or scope for everyone's needs. It is difficult for the audience to assess
how reliable and balanced the content of the presentation is, when faced with
the single view of an enthusiastic expert.

## The workshop

A workshop is a good format for the exchange of ideas and experiences in a relatively new area. It encourages interaction and discussion in response to a short, targeted expert input if it is run well. A workshop relies on the participants being willing to contribute and think out how what they have heard from the expert applies to their situation and justify why or why not they might adopt or adapt what they have heard or worked out, for themselves or their teams. A workshop sometimes follows a didactic lecture giving the audience an opportunity to think the topic through and challenge the speaker's points or views. As a stand alone event it is common for the workshop leader to give a short presentation to launch the subject and areas for discussion. Sometimes the workshop leader acts as an instructor and responds to questions throughout the session. More usually at a conference (see Chapter 7) the purpose of a workshop is to bring conference delegates together from different settings or backgrounds to share their experiences and good practice – then the workshop leader is mainly in a facilitator role.

Sometimes a workshop may be one in a series of learning activities for a cohort of students. Unless you are acting as a consultant or a guest facilitator on a one-off basis, that sort of linked series of workshops or ones that are integral to a particular course are outside the scope of this chapter.

## Ad hoc *teaching*

Much of your teaching may take place in a busy clinical setting, during work time. The learner may ask you for an explanation that refers to their experience as it occurs to them. So in that case you must think on your feet without the luxury of reading up about the subject beforehand or preparing visual aids. Even so, it is possible to prepare for such teaching encounters by having a framework or process in mind that can be used as required, so that it really is not as *ad hoc* a teaching episode as it might superficially appear to be.

# What does this style mean?

> One-off teaching is impersonal, flexible, self confident, self contained, resourceful, centred more on the purpose of teaching than learners' needs, discontinuous.

It could mean that you prefer the more impersonal relationship of lecturer to many learners than the closer working with learners in small groups or the more direct teacher-learner relationship of a tutorial. Although a formal lecture format can be somewhat rigid, effective presenters are still flexible and creative. If there is only you, one room and fifty learners expecting a presentation from you, you will still have flexibility about what audio-visual equipment you use (for example, film clips, PowerPoint presentation, or no audio-visual equipment etc.), the variety afforded by interactive discussions or the content and style of handouts. Even in a lecture theatre it is possible to intersperse discussions, asking people to turn to their neighbours and consider points you have raised.

Consultants or guest teachers who are external to the organisation, may be commissioned to teach on a one-off basis. They may be employed for their expertise in specific areas which the teaching establishment does not have; or because the organisation does not have sufficient teachers on its staff, and paying consultants is more economic than employing regular teachers. Such consultants rarely know those they are teaching, may only have a second-hand knowledge of the learners' needs or preferences, and will be unlikely to follow up with the learners at a later date. They may be more fixed on the commissioning organisation's priorities and needs than those of the learners – after all that is their commission. If this is you, then you must be relatively self contained and self confident to be teaching strangers with whom you have no prior relationship, making your learning relevant to them from hearsay or driving home their employers' messages, by sticking to the details of your commission. You must be flexible and able to adapt your materials and main messages to different audiences. Of course once you are in front of your learners, you can ask them what they want or know already, but your flexibility and capacity to vary your script will be limited by what is possible in a short time frame, in accordance with your commission, and very likely with limited scope to change – your format of delivery, your supporting materials etc.

On the other hand, *ad hoc* teaching will demand that you are flexible and resourceful to take advantage of teaching opportunities as they crop up in the workplace and match your input to the needs of the individual or small group of learners. You will be picking up cues about what learners' views and misunderstandings are. You will not have the opportunity for a full blown needs assessment so will be assessing learners' needs in a sensitive and continual way, partly intuitively.

## Is this style really you?

How you got into teaching might influence the format you usually use. It may be that someone whose main experience has been receiving lectures at school or university, or is accustomed to get managerial type diktats, opts for a lecture format when they teach because they are familiar with that format or because it is what their learners expect. As a new teacher you may not realise how autonomous you are in selecting the most appropriate method of delivery of your teaching. So although you can give lectures, there may be other formats which you could employ and feel comfortable to be teaching in, with which you have little experience. You will need to experiment with different types of teaching formats in supported situations and reflect on your own preferred style as a result.

If you crave feedback from students, the pay back of seeing them develop over time and the value of developing relationships with them may mean that this one-off style will not be for you, except on an occasional basis.

# Making the most of this as your preferred style

The trick is to match your level of delivery with the same level of self direction that the learner has reached, and try to challenge them in their learning as appropriate, depending on the subject matter.

### In respect of the lecture

An unresponsive audience can unnerve the most experienced lecturer or teacher. People behave differently when being taught in a one-to-one situation from when they are attending a lecture as one of a large number of people, or participating in a workshop.[1] In normal conversation the listener actively supports and encourages the speaker by non-verbal signs, making a suggestion if the speaker is lost for a word and synchronising facial expressions and body posture with what the speaker is saying. When a lecturer addresses a large audience not only is that supportive interaction not there, but the audience behaviour may put the speaker off. When you are standing in front of a tiered lecture theatre full of people, their stares can seem like a threat rather than the facial expressions of concentration which they might be, and their uninhibited comfort movements such as head-propping, shuffling and yawning might be mistakenly interpreted as boredom and disrespect which they may not be. It has been described as 'diffusion of responsibility' with 'no one responsible for supporting and providing feedback to the speaker, who may feel, from the lack of apparent response as if he or she is throwing stones into treacle.'[1]

When audiences are primed to put lecturers off by appearing to be inattentive, the presenter performs less well than when audiences are primed to appear supportive and interested. To some extent, audiences should take responsibility for the quality of the lecture they receive. The message for you as a one-off teacher is to expect this type of behaviour, and either resolve not to be put off or take it personally and press on regardless despite little feedback or support, or actively engage the audience by asking questions, triggering discussion, setting challenges and using other interactive techniques.

Help the audience to follow your train of thought and argument by setting out your talk as an introduction, a main theme in the body of the talk with a final summary or conclusion. Let the audience know what to expect when you are introducing your presentation: 'Say what you are going to say, say it and then repeat what you said' as is often recommended. Try not to fall into the traps given in Box 8.1. Find out exactly who will be in the audience and their likely levels of knowledge and experience. Arrive early enough at the lecture venue to set up any audiovisual material and ensure that they are positioned correctly and you know how to operate any equipment – if you are unfamiliar with the venue and layout as a one-off teacher. Take your own equipment with you so you are self-resourced as far as possible (blu tack, pointer, handouts, pens etc.). Have some water standing by if you are a nervous speaker.

Let the audience know before you start whether you will take questions of clarification during your lecture or whether you prefer they keep their questions to the end of your talk.

> **Box 8.1 Traps to avoid when giving a lecture.**
>
> Don't:
> - misjudge your audience or students by either assuming too much or too little prior knowledge
> - deliver your teaching in the wrong way – too fast, too boring, too challenging or use humour inappropriately
> - use the wrong format for the learners – a prescriptive lecture when interaction is required
> - be unfamiliar with the lecture theatre layout and have to delay your presentation whilst you sort out the lighting, seating arrangements, ventilation or audio-visual equipment
> - be too quiet, too quick or speak with too much of an accent for the learner to hear your words clearly
> - deliver the lecture so that the content is difficult to understand and the learners leave the lecture ill informed about the subject or more confused than they were before!
> - have learning outcomes that are irrelevant, or unimportant to the learners and do not match the students' preferences or needs
> - focus on the organisation's priorities to the exclusion of those of the learners, who then switch off if the content of your talk seems to be irrelevant or repetitive.

## In respect of the stand alone workshop:

You might as the workshop leader:

- have different expectations about the workshop topic and content from the workshop participants
- assume that the participants have too much or too little prior knowledge
- take too long in delivering your initial presentation to launch the workshop so that the subsequent time for discussion and group work is insufficient for the task and the workshop turns into a lecture format
- deviate from the advertised content or learning outcomes if your initial presentation is not strictly relevant to the workshop and is more of an opportunity for you to present your views rather than meet the needs of workshop participants
- have an unsuitable room for the workshop – for example it is too small for the number of small groups that are run. If you are given a tiered lecture theatre for running the workshop it will be difficult trying to facilitate an interactive discussion.

So improve by:

- choosing a title for your workshop that is explicit and unambiguous so that potential participants are less likely to be misled about what it will cover

- ensuring that the abstract of the workshop you submitted for potential participants to read prior to the session accurately reflects the scope, content, depth, and challenges of the workshop session, giving realistic backgrounds of you as leader and any other facilitators
- having a preliminary meeting with other workshop facilitators, to agree a consistent approach to the workshop, understanding the learning objectives and expected outcomes, agreeing roles and responsibilities and timing.
- planning and keeping to a workshop timetable. Wear a watch and either keep an eye on it or place it in a prominent position so that you and the other speakers or facilitators can see the time too. As leader sit where you can catch the eye of other contributors if they run over time
- finding out who is likely to be in the audience and their prior knowledge
- letting the organiser know what the upper limit of numbers is for your workshop prior to the event
- producing sufficient copies of handouts so that participants can remind themselves easily about the nature of the task in hand
- arranging for a flip chart to be available for each small group with plenty of paper on each flip chart trestle
- keeping small group reporters to time and focused on presenting the discussion of their tasks
- rounding up the final plenary discussion of the workshop with a conclusion based on the small group discussions that relates back to the objectives of the workshop.

### In respect of ad hoc teaching

The sequence described in Chapter 6 for the five microskills of a one minute teacher is also applicable here to help you to assess, instruct, and give feedback more efficiently whilst on the move.[2]

## Improving this style if it is your least preferred style

Although you may not choose to be a one-off teacher as you prefer continuity, it may be thrust upon you at any stage in your career as a teacher. You might have to fill in for a teaching colleague who is sick and take over their teaching commitment with little notice. You might be invited to give a guest lecture because of your expertise in a particular field. You could be forced to act as a paid consultant for the sake of income generation. And there are always opportunities for *ad hoc* teaching in your everyday life.

If you are a reluctant one-off teacher, you will have to steel yourself for the relatively lonely role of teacher. Go as far as you can in identifying the learners' needs – maybe extrapolating from other teaching you have done with similar groups. Compare those needs with your commission, and try to think of ways that you can address both the commission and what you perceive to be learners' needs if they are different.

Prepare well so that you are confident about the content of your talk and can answer likely questions readily. Take the resources with you that you will need so that you are not thrown by the organisers being inadequately prepared.

As you are a one-off teacher, it will be more difficult for you to get feedback about your performance in lecturing or running a stand alone workshop than when your teaching is integral to a planned course. One way to find out how good you are is overhearing others' conversations – in the toilets, at the next table etc. An evaluation of a learning event might pick up participants' opinions of your delivery and its effects if phrased constructively and searchingly and not focused on relatively trivial details – say the learning environment or joining instructions. A follow-up evaluation several weeks or months later might gauge the extent to which those who listened to your lecture or attended your workshop applied what you taught them, made changes or adopted the essence of your teaching. Multisource feedback is a good way to hear from colleagues, students, managers etc. about your performance, and could be organised to get their perspectives about your *ad hoc* teaching. Or ask a colleague whose opinion you value to sit in the audience of your lecture and give you specific feedback about how you did.

The more you can build up your confidence by any personal management techniques, and yet still retain humility as a teacher so that you try your best to detect learners' needs and preferences and match them whilst sticking to your overall commission, the more effective you will be as a one-off teacher.

## References

1    Neill S. In the stare of ravens. *The Times Higher*. 1999; June 11: 33.

2    Gordon K, Meyer B, Irby D. *The One Minute Preceptor: five microskills for clinical teaching*. Seattle: University of Washington; 1996.

# Chapter 9

# Developing your teaching style and techniques

*Ruth Chambers*

It is important to remember the effect that the teacher has on the learner. Just as the learner has a favoured learning style, the teacher has a preferred teaching style. Your teaching style has a powerful effect on the dynamics of their learning experience and you should adapt it or adopt other styles that are appropriate to the purpose of your teaching, accordingly.

Your appearance and voice are vitally important as well as what you say and your teaching style. Your gestures and body language should be in harmony with your voice and the messages of your presentation, and not be distracting.

You will have developed your teaching style by a mix of what comes naturally to you, and from your experience. There may have been some particular role models whom you have admired who have influenced your style. You might have unconsciously tried to emulate a teacher who you have found inspiring in the past, or purposely avoided being like a teacher with an off putting style. You might have a quiet, introverted personality and tend towards the all-round flexible and adaptable teacher. Or you may be an extrovert and enjoy the big conference teaching style. How you perform as a teacher will have been influenced by the training and feedback you received when preparing for your teaching role. If you are a health professional, the nature of your discipline may have a bearing on your teaching style; doctors may adopt a dominating style and expect to be in charge; whereas nurses and allied health professionals might be more learner-centred from the nature of their professional training and everyday practice.

Your ability to vary your teaching style according to the learners' needs and the purpose of the learning activity will depend on how insightful you are as a person. You should have become more self-aware of the nature of the style you are using and how effective it is, from continuing reflection on your teaching prowess over the years, in response to feedback and evaluation. You can only perform well though when the teaching environment supports you as a competent teacher. Non-work worries may impinge on your performance and awareness of your teaching style – such as health or money worries, working in unfamiliar settings, or when generally harassed.

There will be some teaching styles that come naturally to you, whilst others may make you feel uncomfortable. Make the most of those you are good at;

and practise using the other teaching styles for delivering learning when there is minimal pressure and you can get feedback on how you perform.

## Matching your teaching style to students' learning styles

If you know what your preferred teaching style is you should be more aware as to whether it suits the learning style and needs of your learners. Then you should be able to swop or adapt your teaching style to engage with them more effectively and hopefully have more impact on their gain in knowledge, skills and better attitudes. Well that theory makes good sense anyway. If you are to adapt your teaching style to their learning styles and needs, and to the nature of the topic you are teaching or circumstances you are in, then you need to be optimally aware of your teaching style preferences, and how you can switch styles to order.

Initially you should be aware of your own preferred learning style. For example, you may be a person with a reflector-theorist learning pattern. If you have a trainee who is an activist, they may not respond to the way you emphasise your ideas, principles, maps and models of things. They will want to get on with the task and have a go at new experiences; they may get bored easily and want to move on to learn even more new things. Unless you realise what is going on you may not realise why you and the trainee do not gel. So adopting an all-round flexible and adaptable teaching style, or maybe the sensitive student teacher style, should work better for that trainee, even if your tendency or experience is to be a straight facts no nonsense teacher. It will take self-awareness, feedback from others, and practice for you to be able to adopt or adapt different teaching styles to match the purpose of the learning you are delivering and the preferences or needs of the trainee or nature of the topic.

There are four main approaches to tailoring your teaching to an individual learner's needs:

1 **matching**. Introverts do better with well-structured situations, so a straight facts no nonsense teaching style might suit these type of learners. Extroverts do better with less structured situations – so the all-round flexible and adaptable teaching style would fit well with extrovert learners

2 **allowing choice**. Since learners come from a range of backgrounds and have different ways of learning, and varying aims you should aim for flexibility in your teaching. So the all-round flexible and adaptable teacher should be good here. It may be that a one-off teaching style is useful too where you take advantage of opportunities to teach as they crop up and can tailor your style and content to the specific episode of teaching

3 **providing several different methods of learning on the same course**. This way students can mix and match. They will always find something that suits them. The all-round flexible and adaptable teaching

style fits well here too. The sensitive student-centred teacher will craft their teaching to the various learning styles of the group of learners and specific needs of individual learners. The content might include coverage of factual material where the official curriculum teaching style has a place to cover formal content. An adaptable and experienced teacher should be able to deliver their teaching in various teaching styles. A rigid teacher with a one-only teaching style would be better to work as one of a group of teachers and facilitators to provide a variety of styles that can deliver the several different methods of learning required. The big conference teaching style could be useful too to provide variety, and it might be relevant to include one or more big plenary lectures as an essential format or desirable option for learners as part of their course

4 **independent study**. Complete freedom to study gives good results especially with more mature students. The all-round flexible and adaptable teacher will cope well here.

## Motivation

The effectiveness of your teaching will not just be dependent on your style and content. Motivation will be key too. That is, yours as a teacher to adopt or adapt your teaching style to match the purpose and learners' needs and your ability to motivate learners through adopting a teaching style that is effective. Motivation has been defined as 'that within the individual, rather than without, which incites him or her to action'.[1] Motivation may be positive or negative.

With **positive** motivation your learners will be keen to learn more about a subject because of your skill as an inspiring teacher, because the subject interests them a great deal or they can see the relevance to their future career progress. With **negative** motivation the learners may do things because of the fear of failure or punishment or other adverse things that could happen to them if they do not do something.

Positive motivation tends to leads to deeper understanding and better long term learning than negative methods, which can lead to superficial learning that is often forgotten.

## Matching your style to the teaching format

As you plan to meet your learners' needs and educational objectives you will broaden the range of teaching methods and learning strategies that you can offer them as good teachers do, see Box 9.1. In healthcare there are opportunities for all types of learning sessions, some of which are *ad hoc*, such as those by the bedside or in the out-patient clinic. All however can be planned, or prepared for, to a greater or lesser extent. The type of teaching is dictated to an extent by what resources are available.

---

**Box 9.1 A good teacher will. . .**

- understand the learner's needs
- set appropriate learning objectives
- prepare well so that the context and content is clear and focused
- match the educational methods with those objectives
- stimulate the learner
- challenge the learner
- interest the learner
- involve the learner
- encourage the learner – with positive feedback
- use a style of delivery that suits the learner's needs
- evaluate the teaching and the learning
- refine future teaching in light of evaluation
- be a life-long learner.

---

In considering which teaching method to use, you will be asking yourself the following questions:

- what am I trying to achieve, what are my objectives?
- what are the learners' objectives?
- is this the best way of achieving them?
- what other ways are there of achieving them?
- what are the strengths of the way I have chosen?
- what are the potential weaknesses that I will have to be on the guard for as facilitator?
- how will I know that this way is the most appropriate way – for me and my learners?
- how will I assess whether the objectives have been achieved?

Some teaching styles fit better than others with the various approaches to teaching and methods of learning. See if you agree with the teaching styles that we suggest best fit the methods of learning that follow.

## How comfortable are teachers with different styles in a variety of teaching and learning formats?

The examples below describe various formats of teaching and learning. We go on to suggest that teachers with specific kinds of teaching styles may feel more comfortable with certain types of teaching and learning.

### Problem based learning

Problem based learning (PBL) reverses the traditional approach to teaching and learning. It starts with individual examples or problems, through the consideration of which learners develop general principles and concepts that they can generalise to other situations. It can foster deep learning, requires students to activate prior learning and integrate new learning with it and can develop life-long learning skills and generic competencies such as collaboration.

Working through PBL scenarios:

1  define learning objectives in advance
2  problems should be appropriate to the stage of the curriculum and the level of learner understanding
3  scenarios should be relevant to practice
4  problems should be presented in context to encourage integration of knowledge
5  scenarios should present cues to stimulate discussion and encourage learners to seek an explanation
6  the problem should be of sufficient depth to prevent too early resolution
7  students should be actively engaged in searching for information.

What kinds of teaching style will match the delivery of problem based learning?

• An all-round flexible and adaptable teacher as they will be using all aspects of work and the health environment in setting and solving the PBL topic.
• The straight facts no nonsense teacher as they might focus on the specific knowledge and skills the learner(s) need to resolve a particular situation.

## Computer supported learning

The advantages of online learning are that they give access to a huge amount of information, linking resources in different formats. Such learning allows and supports flexible delivery, distance learning, workplace based learning. Learners can follow the course materials at their own pace, independently, actively and in a way that suits their learning needs. Interactivity, attractive animations and simulations can be built into course materials as easily as less stimulating, traditional materials.

Discussion forums (email, video-conferencing, live lectures, virtual learning environments) can be set up for learner support, collaboration and development. Self-assessments can be built in for students to monitor their own progress – giving quick feedback and freeing up tutors from excessive individual involvement.

What kinds of teaching style will match the composition and delivery of online learning?

• An all-round flexible and adaptable teacher as they will make the most of this flexible format of learning in terms of variety in timing, setting, diversity of learners, application, etc.
• The straight facts no nonsense teacher as they will enjoy the opportunity for relaying clear facts in a logical way, though they may not be as comfortable with the discussion forums as with the composition and assessment of the online learning.

- The one-off teacher as the part they play may be in the composition of the materials without necessarily providing any subsequent support for learning.

## Teaching a practical skill

The teaching of a practical skill is an exercise both in imparting a new skill to a learner as well as an opportunity for discussion on and around the topic in question. Time is often limited and therefore it is appropriate to ensure that an adequate knowledge base has been covered in advance of the session, e.g. anatomy of the region in surgery.

The three basic elements of a practical teaching session are:

1 preparation
2 procedure
3 summary.

What kinds of teaching style will match the teaching of a practical skill?

- The straight facts no nonsense teacher as they can demonstrate the practical skills in recommended ways, though they may not be comfortable with students questioning their recommended approach.
- The one-off teacher as the part they play is to teach the skill so that it is a complete episode of teaching.
- The sensitive student-centred teacher as they may craft the teaching of the practical skill on a one to one basis using an apprentice-like mode.

## Small group teaching

Small groups are a good format to encourage the learners to interact, explore and develop ideas. You might run a small group following after a lecture to allow the learners to debate the points they have just heard, the extent to which they apply them to their own circumstances and how they could change their practice at work or their personal behaviour. Or a small group might be a forum for the exchange of different ideas to help the members learn from each other by sharing tips and experiences that stimulate reflection and forward thinking. Small group work encourages learners to develop their thinking and challenge pre-conceived beliefs; it is often more effective than more passive types of teaching in stimulating learners to think independently.

If attitudes and feelings are involved rather than new clinical facts, then well balanced small group discussions will help individual learners think through the topic and its implications after, or instead of, a didactic lecture. Small group work promotes critical and logical thinking as part of a problem solving approach. The format helps group members to understand why others hold different views and what makes them tick.

Small group work is usually based on a task that is wide enough to encourage the learners to own and develop the topic themselves, but focused enough to restrict the ensuing discussions to the matter in hand. In small group work it is the learners who are key to the subsequent discussion rather than the facilitator whose opinions are of lesser or no importance.

What kinds of teaching style will match the delivery of small group work?

- The sensitive student-centred teacher as they may set up and guide the small group topics and discussions so the participants consider attitudes and behaviour and feelings.
- The all-round flexible and adaptable teacher as small group teaching will be a method they can latch onto between other teaching approaches – such as after a lecture, over a period of time for development, to build a team, or take forward a project plan.

## Handouts

A handout should capture the key points of your talk but need not be too comprehensive as those who are particularly interested in the topic can follow up your session with private reading. Include a reading list or references to key literature or sources of further information. Credit other people's work, giving full references.

What kinds of teaching style will fit with utilising handouts?

- The straight facts no nonsense teacher as they just need to relay the facts, and there is no potential for any extra details.
- The big conference teacher as the handout can supplement their presentation and give them further prestige when readers appreciate that the references cited indicate their associated work.

## Injecting humour

You could use humour to liven up a meeting and encourage collaboration, or provide a different style of learning that should appeal to activists. Do not try to be funny if telling jokes makes you quake or you are hopeless at delivering the punch line. The jokes could be linked to the health field, and chosen

---

**Box 9.2 Using humour to relay your teaching.**

It has been statistically proven that birthdays are good for you – the more you have, the longer you'll live.

One third of car accidents involve drivers who have been drinking alcohol excessively. Thus if two-thirds of drivers in car accidents were sober, we should encourage drivers to drink more alcohol. Discuss!

Treatment for a bad cough? Take a large dose of laxatives and then you will be too afraid to cough!

Life is sexually transmitted.

Health is merely the slowest possible rate at which you can die.

so that they will not cause offence. They might be associated with the topic of your talk or learning session. Look at those in Box 9.2 for starters. They should make learners think about the underlying meaning, though phrased in a humorous way.

You could select a cartoon that has no title and invite your learners to dream up an appropriate heading or a relevant caption – using humour. Or, choose a cartoon or picture of a person/people doing something or thinking something – draw in one or more speech bubbles for the participants to complete. The essence of the cartoon or picture should be relevant to the theme of your learning event. Ask the participants to work in pairs or small groups on the task. You could ask them to report back by shouting out their contributions, writing on their suggestions and pinning them up on a board for participants to look at, at their leisure, or writing their responses on post-its and sticking those up under a replica of the cartoon for general inspection. Working with others will generate more ideas and create laughter as suggestions are exchanged and people become more outrageous. It will lighten the atmosphere and get everyone ready for the subsequent learning session.

What kinds of teaching style will fit with injecting humour into teaching?

- The one-off teacher as they might use humour to establish immediate rapport.
- The big conference teacher as they might start their presentation with a humorous anecdote in their warm up or interspersed throughout their talk to keep the audience awake and engaged.
- The all-round flexible and adaptable teacher who is ready to try any format or technique that engages learners and increases the impact of their teaching.

### Interactive exercises e.g. draw a personal map of support mechanisms[2]

You could use this technique with a group of people who have been meeting regularly and feel comfortable sharing feelings. Alternatively you can use it when teaching on a one to one basis.

Ask the participant(s) to draw themselves in the middle of a piece of plain paper. Then they should draw little pictures around the edge of the paper to represent all the sources of support in their life – people, things, situations, environment etc. (see the example in Figure 9.1). They can then add drawings of what other sources of support they have used in the past but not employed for a while, and what extra sources of support they would like to have, maybe in a different coloured ink. They will link each picture to themselves in the centre of the page. Then they should draw in the barriers that stop them from using these sources of support across the line linking that particular source. Lastly, they should consider which are their strongest sources of support, those they would like to enhance, the nature of the barriers that stop them from making more of their sources of support, and what is missing. This exercise helps people to review the extent and type of sources of support that exist for them at work or outside work.

What kinds of teaching style will fit with setting interactive exercises?

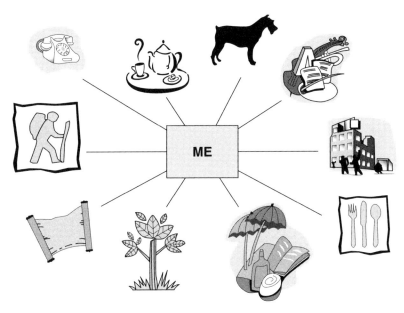

**Figure 9.1** A personal support map. (Reproduced from Chambers R, Schwartz A, Boath E. *Beating Stress in the NHS*. Oxford: Radcliffe Medical Press; 2003.)

- An all-round flexible and adaptable teacher as they can encourage learners to draw on a wide range of sources of support in their home and working lives.
- The sensitive student-centred teacher as they can enable discussion of the personal support maps, feeling comfortable when emotions and feelings inevitably come to the fore.

## Using visual props

**Photographs**: the use of photographs can trigger general and then in-depth discussions about health or other issues illustrated in the photographs, the societal and environmental factors likely to be associated with the pictures and alternative interventions that could be tried. The visual imagery will appeal to everyone and prove the saying 'a picture is worth a thousand words'. Using photographs will trigger lateral thinking when looking at a topic in-depth for new solutions or innovations. Used early on in small group work it helps the participants to start talking and begin to gel. Later on, in small or large group work, it can waken up a fatigued audience by changing the pace and style of the learning event and introducing new ideas. Everyone should be engaged by the right picture. You can expect previously disinterested or non-contributing members of the group to become engaged in discussion.

**Symbols**: some teachers use symbols to represent the topics, feelings, knowledge etc. that they are talking about or wanting learners to dwell on. This might include pictures of mountains, or buildings (modern, in disrepair etc.), it might be national flags, a style of salute or dress.

**Picture with deliberate mistakes:** you could use this pictorial exercise in a workshop to stimulate the learners, encourage their collaboration, or test their knowledge. You can give everyone a copy of a picture (e.g. see Figure 9.2) to mark the deliberate mistakes (hazards in our example) and then discuss their conclusions as a group. Different people will spot some or most of the mistakes you have depicted. Bring everyone together and pool observations and the team should realise that their collaboration has identified many more of the hazards (if not all) that exist. A topic such as 'health and safety', as in our example, should be appropriate when disparate members of a team are attending of varying seniority – to provide a topic for which they are mainly at the same level; or a multidisciplinary mix of learners.

In this example the illustration shows a rather disorganised workplace. Try to spot the hazards – they might occur in any office workplace. See below to find the answers.

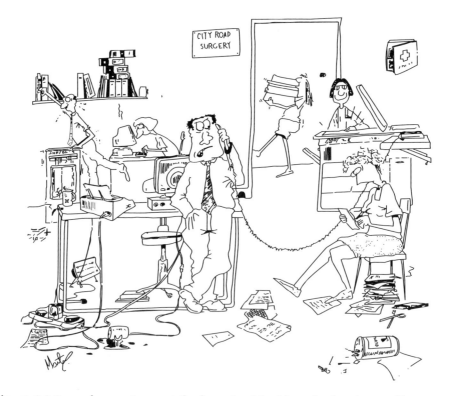

**Figure 9.2** Example exercise: spot the hazards of health and safety in an office environment.[3]

Answers to example given for Figure 9.2. Did you spot the hazards in the fictitious premises? We found thirty:

• sharps box on floor spilling out needles
• coffee cup spilling its contents on the floor
• coffee mug by the printer has been repaired, so is dangerous

- trailing wires from the phone and computer and printer
- overloaded adapter with many wires plugged into the socket
- open electric fire without a guard
- electric fire is near to a trailing lead
- unattended cigarette butt burning on the table
- secretary's cigarette lying on top of a pile of papers by her chair
- scissors lying open on the floor
- electric lead to computer frayed in the middle
- computer chair propped up on books, as a wheel is missing
- printer almost falling off the edge of the table
- urgent notice lying on the floor
- private letter lying on the floor
- secretary sitting just below the telephone shelf, likely to hit her head when she gets up
- poor posture of the secretary
- poor posture of the computer operator in the background
- dangerous pile of files on a shelf
- coffee mug poised on a high shelf above the computer operator – hot contents might tip over her
- man over-reaching for books on a high shelf
- man in the background poorly balanced and in danger of catching his fingers and tie in the shredder
- shredder has spilt waste paper on the floor – fire hazard
- letters on the floor by the secretary are a fire hazard
- papers and letters on the floor create a potential hazard which might trip up a passer-by
- lady in the background carrying an awkward and heavy load
- photocopier lid is open causing possible eye strain hazard to the operator
- first aid box has an open door
- mouse hole – there may be vermin
- overcrowded room – threatens the privacy of confidential phone calls.

What kinds of teaching style will match the inclusion of visual props in teaching?

- An all-round flexible and adaptable teacher will feel confident about using various visual materials and interactive exercises to stimulate learning in any way that works.
- The one-off teacher will see that the visual props help them to deliver self-contained items of teaching in an engaging way.

## One to one learning

The tutorial is the formal setting for one to one learning but valuable learning can also take place informally in the workplace, at the bedside in the consulting room etc. Learning opportunities can be fleeting moments and should be grasped firmly as they arise – this may be following a ward round, in the ward office or in the common room after a general practice surgery, or in the car between domiciliary visits. Look out for opportunities – seize the day!

It is the learning environment and the climate generated that is all-important. The learning will be greater if the room is comfortable and free from interruptions. Time must be protected. The aims and objectives of the one to one session need to be planned and based on the needs of the learner as for any other learning activity. Feedback should be positive and constructive. Tutorials are ideal opportunities for role play or watching videotapes of the learner's (or teacher's) consultations in a safe environment. Similarly, in-depth discussion of a specific patient's problems using random case, or critical event, analyses are also ideal subjects for the intimate environment of a one to one tutorial.

Many factors may impair the one to one educational experience. The quality of the learning experience depends on you as a teacher but also the commitment and attitude of your learner.

What kinds of teaching style fit with one to one learning?

- The official formal curriculum teacher, if regular tutorials are a required part of delivering a course or training programme. The tutorial will probably follow a set template.
- The sensitive student-centred teacher as they will use the tutorial situation to discuss emotions and feelings to encourage the learner to give their perspective and develop new insights.

# References

1   Peyton JWR. *Teaching and Learning in Medical Practice*. Rickmansworth: Manticore Europe; 1998.

2   Chambers R, Mohanna K, Chambers S. *Survival Skills for Doctors and their Families*. Oxford: Radcliffe Medical Press; 2003.

3   Chambers R, Hawksley B, Smith G, *et al*. *Back Pain Matters in Primary Care*. Oxford: Radcliffe Medical Press; 2001.

# Chapter 10

# Evaluating teaching sessions: is your teaching style effective?

*Kay Mohanna*

Educational evaluation is:

> a systematic approach to collection, analysis and interpretation of information about any aspect of conceptualisation, design, implementation and utility of educational programmes. Evaluation measures the teaching. It is not the same as discussing a learner's progress with them (appraisal) or measuring what students have learnt (assessment). Results of appraisal and assessment processes as well as learner feedback however can be incorporated into evaluations.[1]

There is a risk with evaluation of healthcare teaching practice that the essential elements are the hardest to define and measure. Aspects such as transfer of learning into the workplace and impact on healthcare outcomes, are overlooked. Attributes that we can all define are measured and we count those aspects which we can see. So evaluation processes based on learner feedback might address questions such as did the lecture keep to time, did the teacher set clear objectives, were the teaching activities aligned with the objectives, did the students express satisfaction or did they do well on their tests?

A report into the effectiveness of continuing professional development observed that:

> In complex fields of practice there is a risk that [evaluation] highlights the readily measurable, over-emphasising detail, rather than promoting essential aspects of competence. In this way teaching practice is trivialised through [evaluation] that fails to support competence development.[2]

This book is about promoting effectiveness in teaching through defining and developing our preferred teaching style. We recognise that teacher differences exist and are as influential on the learning process as learner difference. If we want to look at how effective we are as teachers, it is essential that we look at that difference in style as it affects that most important variable – learner competence.

## The evaluation cycle[3]

Evaluation is a vital component of the educational process. It should be considered right at the beginning of the planning stage of an educational activity so that we know what questions we need to ask to be able to say: 'did we achieve what we set out to do?' For example, consider the evaluation cycle outlined below.

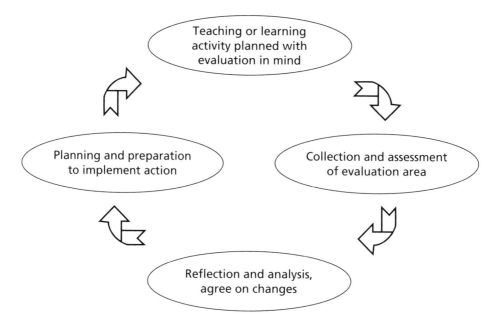

**Figure 10.1** Evaluation cycle.

In 1987 Kirkpatrick described a hierarchy of evaluation, or four levels on which to focus our questions,[4] and these have recently been adapted for use in health education.[5] Table 10.1 below considers the four levels that apply throughout the whole range of evaluative techniques and situations.

As a general rule we are looking for mechanisms of evaluation that look at higher order outcomes: what impact is our teaching having on the day to day practice of our learners?

In Chapter 2 we described our development of the SETS tool. At the end of that chapter we gave you the opportunity to discover what your teaching style was by working through the questionnaire for yourself, so by now you may know what your preferred teaching styles are. This chapter gives you the opportunity to evaluate your success in teaching by specific reference to the characteristics we have defined as part of that style. We hope this chapter will help you look at those aspects of each style that can be evaluated and whether those activities you prefer as a teacher, are also the ones you are most effective in.

**Table 10.1** Evaluating educational activities: the four levels.[5]

| | Evaluation of | Measure | Participant |
|---|---|---|---|
| 1 | **Reaction** | Satisfaction or happiness | What is the participant's response to the programme? |
| 2 | **Learning** | Knowledge or skills acquired Modification of attitudes or perceptions | What did the participant learn? |
| 3 | **Behaviour** | Transfer of learning to workplace | Did the participant's learning affect their behaviour? |
| 4 | **Results** | Transfer or impact on society | Did changes in the participant's behaviour affect their organisation? Were any benefits or problems noted as a result of these changes? |

Remember, the characteristics that we list as part of each style arose out of the self-reported activities of over 130 healthcare teachers in our original work. Having determined which style you *prefer*, you may well start to see such patterns in your work. It is up to you however to evaluate whether in fact you *do them well.* It is of course possible that circumstance and your teaching opportunities have in fact moulded the type of teacher you have become and there might be scope for you to develop other attributes through self evaluation.

## The all-round flexible and adaptable teacher

> This teacher can use lots of different skills, can teach both peers and juniors, and is very aware of the whole environment both in teaching and of the learners.

The skill of being a great teacher is in knowing how to respond to learners in ways that effectively address the differences between them and to be able to facilitate learning in a variety of ways that also takes into account differences in subject matter and setting. To evaluate this type of all-rounder, we need an evaluation structure that can be used in any situation in which the teacher might find themselves.

Table 10.2 gives an example of an evaluation form based on Table 10.1.

As we consider each of the other teaching styles below, we will look at situation specific types of evaluation strategy. The all-round flexible teacher can use any of the following methods to look at their effectiveness. If you are able to change the way in which you structure your teaching, so you will also be able to select and apply an appropriate evaluation tool.

**Table 10.2** Evaluation of a teaching session, appropriate for many different settings.

| *Evaluation of:* | *Question* |
| --- | --- |
| **Reaction** | To what extent was this programme/course/workshop/tutorial pitched at the right level for your needs? Please circle one of the numbers that best represents your view |
| | It was pitched at just the right level for my needs |
| | 1    2    3    4    5 |
| | (1 = totally disagree; 5= totally agree) |
| **Learning** | What were the three most important things you learnt today? |
| | A |
| | B |
| | C |
| | What areas for further learning have you identified? |
| | A |
| | B |
| | C |
| **Behaviour** | In what way will you do things differently after today? |
| **Results** | How will you know if these things you do differently have affected outcomes in your workplace? |

## The student-centred sensitive teacher

This teacher is very student-centred, teaches in small groups, with emotions to the fore, using role play and drama, and is not comfortable doing straight presentations.

As we aim to develop high levels of self direction and independence in learners, and equip them with the skills to allow them to continue to develop on their own as lifelong learners, student-centredness has become very popular in healthcare teaching. Setting the learner at the focus of the educational activity allows us to tailor teaching to their needs and respond to individual differences.

The rationale employed by teachers who favour this style of teaching is that healthcare education cannot be a content-based discipline. The curriculum is too wide and the subject matter too fast-changing to allow us to deliver any more than a fraction of all that a practitioner will need once he enters the profession. Rather, we aim to equip learners with the ability to problem solve and adapt in new situations. Not to *know*, but to be able to *find out*. How to do that effectively and efficiently will of course depend on the learning style, preferences and previous experience of the learners.

Clearly there is much that new entrants to the healthcare professions will need to know, but a student-centred teacher chooses to help learners acquire new knowledge, skills and attitudes whilst at the same time developing meta-cognitive skills such as reflective practice, problem solving and critical thinking. So for example the teaching activities will be chosen to allow more group work with time for negotiation and team building to occur along with leadership, resource investigation and creativity.

If you are a student-centred, sensitive teacher, quite unlike the straight facts no nonsense teacher (see section below), you will be comfortable helping students to develop in the affective domain – considering attitudes and professional behaviours. In order to achieve this you will design teaching activities that allow them to discuss and exchange views. At the same time in order to develop knowledge and skills you will design teaching activities around case discussions and consideration of the perspectives of all players in a scenario. You may, for example, develop safe environments where you expect learners to act in role plays.

Evaluation in such a situation can be complex. This type of learning is often achieved best in groups, or for individuals, working over time such as vocational training schemes in general practice for example or apprenticeship learning where the environment is under the control of tutor and trainee over a period of time.

One way to evaluate success in that environment is with a naturalistic approach. Naturalistic evaluation is a model that takes into account participants' definitions of key concerns and issues. The mode of data collection is

---

**Box 10.1 Naturalistic evaluation.**

You are going to be working together as a group for the rest of this term. At the end of the course, we will be interested to find out about your experience and whether you feel your objectives have been met. We are particularly interested in how that happened and any aspects that might have acted as barriers to you achieving your goals.

In your tutorial groups, please define what you consider to be the important aspects of this course by considering the following questions:

1  What are you hoping to achieve in terms of
  – knowledge
  – skills
  – attitudes?
2  How will you know if you have achieved them?
3  How will you measure success?
4  How will you identify features that facilitated your learning?
5  How will you identify barriers to success?

Your lists will be used to form the basis of focus group discussion at the end of the course to see whether a consensus can be reached about the success of the course. You will be asked to appoint a facilitator and scribe for the focus group.

qualitative. It allows the learners to set the investigative agenda and determine the criteria for evaluation. The language that is used and the mode of presenting the findings is intended to be accessible to participants.

A proposed scheme for such an evaluation process is given in Box 10.1.

Such a process needs well-motivated learners who understand the nature of the evaluation. In addition the timing of the focus group discussion in relation to the timing of the activity is an important area to be considered. Self-reported satisfaction with courses fades over time as participants return to work, or enter practice, and find it hard to implement changes arising from what they learnt on the course. Good outcome scores in early evaluation may not therefore be sustained, or achieved, if evaluation is carried out too far from the event but, similarly, less good performance in evaluation later on may give a better overall judgment about the impact of the course.

# The official curriculum teacher

> This teacher is very well prepared as a teacher, is likely to be accredited, is very aware of and teaches to the formal curriculum and follows external targets for teaching.

If this is your preferred teaching style, how could you evaluate aspects of your teaching to maximise outcomes for learners and minimise anxiety for you in your preparation and delivery?

In an attempt to minimise the discomfort that may arise from a feeling of un-preparedness, these teachers are likely to have ensured that they have been trained to teach, and have attended and completed appropriate teaching the teachers courses. As an official curriculum teacher, have you been on a teaching the teachers course? Or are you in fact one of those healthcare teachers who has ended up as a formal teacher by virtue of your seniority or because it is expected of you? If so, it may be that you find teaching more stressful than need be. Simply asking yourself questions about training is a form of evaluation. How well prepared am I to be a teacher? How likely is it that all learners will be satisfied with the type of activities I plan? What do I know about the underlying educational theory of how people learn? Would formal continuing professional development in this area help me to be more comfortable and effective in my role?

Teachers who are comfortable in this style set great store by being well prepared as a teacher. They will have planned and prepared the sessions to be taught well in advance, having all the materials there and being familiar with how to use them. They will know that such preparation fits in with what is meant to be covered in the curriculum.

If you find this style comfortable, then you are less likely to be comfortable with a 'seat of the pants' type of teaching. You may find problem based learning sessions challenging to facilitate requiring, as they do, a much less teacher-centred approach to the educational activity. Ask your learners specific questions that refer to your preferred teaching style.

The official curriculum teacher makes a point of being very familiar with the formal curriculum statements for the teaching and sets clear aims and objectives that they then ensure they can achieve. This teacher is very careful to match their teaching with these curriculum statements, so that the whole curriculum is properly covered. If this is not your preferred teaching style, you are much more likely to be uncomfortable with what you perceive as a restrictive approach to the content of your teaching. Simply recognising this as a difference in style can allow you to challenge yourself and adapt the teaching you organise.

Suggested evaluation strategies to consider if you are an official curriculum teacher are given in Table 10.3.

**Table 10.3** Evaluation of the official curriculum teacher.

| Evaluation of | Question | Outcomes |
|---|---|---|
| **Reaction** | Ask the learners about your facilitation style. You could ask the learners to indicate on a Likert-type scale their answers to the following stems:<br><br>How would you describe the effectiveness of each of the following types of teaching on this course?<br><br>• coaching with immediate feedback<br>• informational lecture<br>• guided discussion<br>• goal-setting activities<br>• seminars<br>• group projects<br>• individual work or self-directed study-group. | Dependent learners or more teacher-centred content might prompt a response that suggests your formal curriculum approach works well and matches with learner style. More independent or self directed learners, or more problem-based content may evoke a response that a less hands-on approach to teaching would be more effective for these learners. You might then adjust the type of activities you provide. |
| **Learning** | Incorporate assessment of learner achievement into your evaluation:<br><br>What proportion of learners achieved the:<br>• knowledge<br>• skills<br>• attitudes<br><br>aimed for in this course? | What did the participants learn?<br><br>Was it a course aiming to increase knowledge? If so were your aims and objectives clear so learners knew what they needed to know?<br><br>Was this a skill based course? If so, were learners given the chance to practise?<br><br>Was it an attitudinal development outcome? If so did learners have a chance to debate with peers and hear opposing views? |

*continued*

**Table 10.3** Continued

| Evaluation of | Question | Outcomes |
| --- | --- | --- |
| | | As a formal curriculum teacher, you may be more comfortable as a source of expert knowledge and less effective at facilitating open discussions. An assessment of learning mapped against a consideration of what you had set out to achieve may give insights into different strategies you might adopt. |
| **Behaviour** | Transfer of learning to workplace:<br><br>The advantage of a formal curriculum is that it clearly lays out content, teaching strategy and intended outcome. One effective evaluation tool would be to audit change in learners' practice in those areas in the teaching programme. Consider a pre-test, post-test design, a method that compares behaviour before and after your intervention. It looks for consistency or 'alignment' between goals, experiences, and outcomes. Behaviours can be measured either by norm-referenced or criterion-referenced tests. | Did the participants' learning affect their behaviour?<br><br>As a formal curriculum teacher you are likely to be very clear on what changes in behaviour you would expect, and be able to recognise it when present in learners after the teaching. The difficulty may be in determining whether it was your intervention that brought about this change. |
| **Results** | Impact of learning.<br><br>What effect has been felt from the change in behaviour your teaching has brought about in learners?<br><br>Results of teaching can be complex. Attributing change to a single intervention by a teacher requires careful planning. However it is possible to audit aspects such as significant event analysis, critical incident reporting and audit of care that will reflect any impact of changed behaviour on care. | Did changes in the participants' behaviour affect their organization? Were any benefits or problems noted as a result of these changes?<br><br>The formal curriculum teacher will be setting teaching activities designed to address specific requirements. Such specific outcomes then, if present, can be considered to be markers of successful transfer and impact of teaching. |

# The straight facts no nonsense teacher

> This teacher likes to teach the clear facts, with straight talking, concentrating on specific skills, and much prefers not to be involved with multi-professional teaching and learning.

So this style describes teachers who prefer to teach the clear facts, in simple language, often distilling the subject to be taught into a small number of key principles. When teaching skills, often these teachers have perfected simple, clear techniques for procedures and can teach them in a logical and step-wise way.

Our research showed that such teachers may not be happy in a multi-disciplinary and multi-professional role, teaching and interacting with other professions within the health service or teaching lay people about medical matters. This may be due to their content-specific approach to modelling knowledge so that it can be delivered in a reproducible way but with little variation in style or room for flexibility or learner difference.

If you fall into this category, you will be a teacher who has thought a lot about the areas that you like to teach, and you will be very clear about the right and wrong answers to questions in these areas. You will probably be highly valued and respected as a skills teacher, within your professional area. An important aspect for you to evaluate will be aspects around learner confidence and their sense of achievement. Do your learners feel confident that they know what the important areas to cover are, that they have identified areas they need to develop or study further, or do they feel confident that they could face an emergency and rely on the grounding you have given them?

You will however probably be quite uneasy teaching in the attitudes domain where there is more room for individual variation in solutions to challenges. As we saw in Chapter 6, if you are involved in teaching about breaking bad news for example, you will have again distilled this down into a series of steps. This will be thoroughly covered but perhaps in rather a mechanistic way not necessarily considering aspects such as the impact of this type of discussion on those engaged in it.

So, what suggestions would we make for evaluation strategies for the straight facts no nonsense teacher? Evaluative questions for participants can be designed around the stages of the educational cycle. Some useful questions are given in Box 10.2:

---

**Box 10.2 Evaluating the straight facts no nonsense teacher.**

**Needs assessment**:
- was the session relevant to you?
- were your needs met?
- what was the extent of needs that were not met?
- were problems solved?

- were some problems left unsolved?
- were any problems not tackled?

**Objectives setting**:
- were the objectives clear?
- were the important aspects included?
- what else did you need to know about?

**Methods**:
- were the methods appropriate e.g. could you read the slides and overheads? how were the handouts?
- was there time for discussions and asking questions?
- was there enough time to practise with and without supervision?

**Assessment**:
- what might you do differently in your practice?
- how might those in your workplace benefit from what you have learnt today?

If you leave free text for comments, sometimes you will get the best suggestion here. But you will need to pose a stem question that is sufficiently inspiring to raise the level of the feedback. Consider:

What suggestions do you have to help this course really make an impact on patient care?

## The big conference teacher

This teacher likes nothing better than to stand up in front of a big audience. This teacher does not like sitting in groups or one to one teaching.

These teachers either have a natural style or have developed themselves to be able to enjoy everyone's attention (or at least tolerate it). They are able to lead, inspire, convey their vision and views, engage others in a confident manner and convince others of their expertise and potential. Many big conference teachers are invited because they are leaders, opinion makers, or experts in their fields. It does not follow that they are good at engaging a large audience. All of us if placed in this position can however follow the rules in Chapter 7 and practise to improve our technique and avoid some of the pitfalls. Whether or not we are comfortable in this role though, we will still need to evaluate our performance to know whether we are good at it.

Frequently, as a speaker at a big conference you will not be able to influence the methods of evaluation used as this will be developed by the organising committee or host. Frequently also, the methods used may not be a full evaluation but rather participants' feedback based on forms placed in conference packs beforehand. The rate of return on these forms varies but may be as low as 15% at big conferences with many sessions. In this case, you need to bear in mind that the feedback may come from quite specific members of the audience – those with a particular point to make – they either really liked you or really did not like you.

So if you want an evaluation of your performance as a big conference teacher, what would a good feedback form look like? Box 10.3 gives an example.

---

**Box 10.3 Evaluation of the big conference teacher.**

**Satisfaction**:
• did this session meet your expectations?
• what went well for you today?
• what could have gone better?

**Knowledge and skills**:
• what do you know now that you didn't know before?
• what helped this learning to occur?
• what got in the way of learning?

**Transfer of skills**:
• what will you do differently in your practice?

**Impact**:
• how will your workplace be affected by what you have learnt in this session?

---

Or how about putting a stamped, self addressed postcard on everyone's seat beforehand. Get them to fill them in when they are back at home or after three months depending which type of feedback you are interested in and ask them to post them to you. You could ask them what message they took home from your talk or what they have implemented back at work, with what effect.

## The one-off teacher

This teacher likes to deliver small self-contained bits of teaching, on a one to one basis, with no props to help and no follow up.

One-off teaching might be in lecture, workshop or *ad hoc* style, and each format will require a different type of evaluation. *Ad hoc* teaching will demand that you are flexible and resourceful enough to take advantage of teaching opportunities as they crop up in the workplace and be able to match your input to the needs of the individual or small group of learners. You will be picking up cues about what learners' views and misunderstandings are 'on the hoof'. You will not have the opportunity for a full-blown needs assessment so will be assessing learners' needs in a sensitive and continual way, partly intuitively. This can make evaluation difficult as you cannot always apply an objectives or outcomes approach. You will need the same flexibility and creativity that you apply to the teaching process to devise an appropriate evaluation process.

What options do we have for evaluating the one-off teacher? You may not want to deliver this exact teaching session again as it may have arisen in response to a particular set of circumstances such as a question from a junior in outpatients, or because you have been asked to stand in for an absent colleague. Or you may be invited to deliver a one-off lecture or run a workshop in a programme devised by a third party. You could consider peer review, a process of observation and feedback from a trusted colleague to give feedback on your strengths as well as help you identify areas to develop. If you are asked to run a workshop or give a lecture for a group of learners for whom you have no ongoing responsibility or continuity, their specific feedback may be complemented by a colleague giving you feedback on the process, rather than the content of your teaching.

Setting up formal or informal peer-feedback on performance can gather important feedback that might otherwise be lost for example in an impromptu teaching setting. Asking a colleague who is around at the time of spontaneous teaching on a ward round for example, allows you to gather feedback that would seem inappropriate to stop and gather from learners.

**Table 10.4** Peer evaluation of teaching.

| Prompts | Strengths | Weaknesses |
|---|---|---|
| Clarity of objectives | | |
| Evidence of planning and organisation | | |
| Methods/approach | | |
| Delivery and pace | | |
| Content (currency, accuracy, relevance, use of examples, level, match to students' needs) | | |
| Student participation | | |
| Use of accommodation and learning resources | | |

Perhaps as a surgeon you are in theatre with an anaesthetist colleague who could act as a peer reviewer and give feedback on how you deal with impromptu teaching as it comes up during an operation. Maybe you can ask a fellow speaker on a day-long programme to give feedback on your session. You will have to develop your own guidelines for how you want to gather feedback and prepare in advance for such opportunities but as you spend time writing your talk for a conference for example, you could also put together a quick handout for a colleague whom you might be able to persuade to critique your work on the day.

Table 10.4 contains an evaluation document adapted from the Higher Education Council for England monitoring forms for university teachers, which you could use.[1]

For further details on different evaluation techniques see also our earlier book where some of the material in this chapter has appeared previously.[1]

# References

1 Mohanna K, Wall D, Chambers R. *Teaching Made Easy*: *a manual for health professionals*. 2nd ed. Oxford: Radcliffe Medical Press; 2004.

2 Grant J, Stanton F. *The effectiveness of continuing professional development*. London: Joint Centre for Education in Medicine; 1999.

3 Wilkes M, Bligh J. Evaluating educational interventions. *BMJ*. 1999; **18**: 1269–72.

4 Kirkpatrick DL. *Evaluating Training Programs: the four levels*. San Francisco: Berrett-Koehler Publishers; 1994.

5 Barr H, Freeth D, Hammick M. *Evaluations of interprofessional education: a United Kingdom review of health and social care*. CAIPE/BERA, 2000.

# Chapter 11

# Building up evidence of your competence as a teacher

*Ruth Chambers*

In the drive to regulate health professionals' standards of practice,[1,2] they must collect and retain information that demonstrates that they meet those standards in their everyday work. If you teach, you need to gather evidence that you are maintaining your competence as a teacher too.

The onus is on you as a professional to show that you are up to date, fit to practise and teach throughout your career. So give some thought to the nature of the evidence that you should collect that reflects the effectiveness of your teaching style as well as your roles and responsibilities as a teacher.

## Demonstrating your competence through a personal portfolio

Pull together a portfolio of evidence of your learning and development as well as your standards of practice or competence. Your portfolio may have multi-uses such as to obtain credits for 'Prior Learning' with higher degree courses at universities as well as to describe your experience and competence. Supporting documents in your portfolio will be useful for your annual appraisal as well as for the basis of your professional revalidation or recertification. Nurse teachers will draw on their portfolio for Post Registration Education and Practice (PREP). Introduced in 1990, PREP was again endorsed by the Nursing and Midwifery Council (NMC) in 2002 and requires nurses to undertake and record their continuing professional development over the three years prior to renewal of their professional registration.[3]

Similarly for doctors, your portfolio should contain an evolving personal development plan and a variety of evidence of competence that matches the headings of *Good Medical Practice*, including teaching and training.[4]

The steps in portfolio based learning are:[5]

- identifying significant experiences as important sources of learning – maybe feedback from those you have taught indicating that your teaching style is, or is not, appropriate

- reflecting on the learning that arose from those experiences – you might discuss that feedback with a teaching colleague and receive their observations too
- demonstrating learning in practice – maybe a second lot of feedback from the same group of learners when you have tried a different teaching style
- analysing the portfolio and identifying further learning needs and ways in which these needs can be met – maybe you try other teaching styles for different settings and circumstances and involve a colleague in peer review.

Analysis of the experiences and learning opportunities in your portfolio should show demonstrable learning outcomes and any further educational plan to meet educational needs or development still outstanding. A mentor or colleague may guide you as you compile and analyse the material in your portfolio, providing another perspective that challenges you to think more deeply about your own attitudes, knowledge or beliefs – as a teacher. Much of the learning emanating from a portfolio is from your individual reflection and self-critique in the analysis stage.

# What is competence?

A good definition of competence is:

> able to perform the tasks and roles required to the expected standard.[6]

You will need to describe the standards expected in the range of tasks and roles you undertake as a teacher and reference the source of standard setting. Consider other people's perspectives too in describing the standards such as those of students, patients or the NHS as a whole.

There is a difference between being competent, and performing in a consistently competent manner. You need to be motivated to perform consistently well and enabled to do so by working within efficient systems and with sufficient resources. There will need to be sufficient numbers of other competent teaching staff and available infrastructure for you to be able to perform consistently well, such as administration to organise the teaching sessions, teaching aids and resources.[7]

You should be competent in most or all the teaching styles we suggest, even if only one or two are your preferred styles. If you have to give a major presentation at a conference, the sensitive student-centred teaching style is unlikely to match the purpose of your talk or the needs and preferences of those in the audience, for instance. But your preference for a one-off teaching style will overlap with the style you need to project when giving a keynote presentation at a conference. Depending on purpose and the content you must cover in your conference presentation, the official formal curriculum teaching style might be relevant in some cases.

## Identifying your learning needs as a teacher

Choose a range of methods to identify your learning needs in your teaching development or delivery, so that you validate the findings of one method by another. For instance, if you are only just starting to consider what your preferred teaching style is, and whether your teaching styles are appropriate for some of your various teaching duties, you might focus on evaluating the effectiveness of your teaching style in one to one, small group and conference situations.

No one method will give you reliable information about the gaps in your knowledge, skills or attitudes or everyday service. It is particularly difficult to determine what it is you 'don't know you don't know' by yourself, yet it is vital that you identify and rectify those gaps. Other people may be able to tell you what you need to learn quite readily. Colleagues from different disciplines could usefully comment on any shortfalls in how your work interfaces with theirs. Learners for whom you are no longer responsible and are therefore no longer under any obligation to you could tell you whether any aspects of your teaching style are off-putting or inappropriate. There may be information you could gather from peer review that could point out those gaps in your knowledge or skills of which you were previously unaware. Seek and accept honest, constructive and timely feedback.

Determine what it is that you 'don't know you don't know' about the effectiveness of your teaching style(s) and ability to teach by:

- asking learners and ex-learners for feedback
- comparing your performance against best practice or that of peers
- comparing your performance against objectives in relation to standards for teaching in your organisation
- asking colleagues from different disciplines about shortfalls in how your work interfaces with theirs.

## Collating evidence about your performance as a teacher

You may decide to use a few selected methods to gather baseline evidence of your performance, focused on your specific area of expertise. You may target other topics or areas at the same time that are relevant to the various sections of the GMC's booklet *Good Medical Practice*.[4] For this type of combined assessment, you might use several of the methods such as:

- constructive feedback maybe organised in a multisource feedback exercise (see Box 11.1) about your teaching styles or delivery from learners, peers or patients (the wider the spread of people giving feedback, the more rounded the picture
- self-assessment, or review by others, using a rating scale to assess your skills and attitudes

- comparison with protocols and guidelines for checking how well procedures are followed and you delivered your teaching accordingly
- audit: various types and applications
- significant event audit relating to teaching and training
- SWOT (strengths, weaknesses, opportunities and threats) analysis of your teaching style(s)
- monitoring access and availability to teaching – how often are your tutorials cancelled due to service needs?
- assessing risk of unsupervised learners for whom you are responsible
- comparing the content of your teaching with that required by professional regulation or legislation
- reviewing teamwork and the share of teaching responsibility
- reflecting on whether you are providing quality educational opportunities
- reflecting on, or evaluating, whether you are providing cost effective educational opportunities.

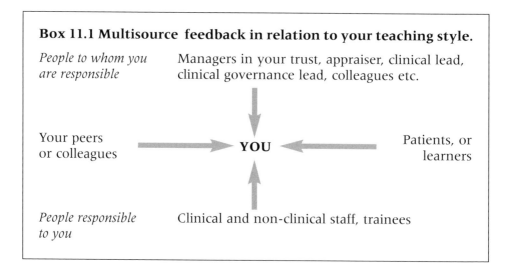

**Box 11.1 Multisource feedback in relation to your teaching style.**

*People to whom you are responsible*  Managers in your trust, appraiser, clinical lead, clinical governance lead, colleagues etc.

Your peers or colleagues  →  **YOU**  ←  Patients, or learners

*People responsible to you*  Clinical and non-clinical staff, trainees

## Learning from significant event audit and making changes

The process of significant event audit or analysis is a good method you could employ to review the effectiveness of your teaching style in particular situations. Think of an incident where you were involved in a significant event and how you used it as a learning opportunity. This might be a dysfunctional tutorial, or very poor feedback after a lecture you gave. This might be due to the content of your teaching, your teaching style or the learning environment. You can review the 'case' and reflect on the sequence of events that led to that critical event occurring. It is likely that there were a multitude of factors leading up to that significant event. How did you respond to it? What learning opportunities did you take from it? Did you shy away from bringing it up with the learner or did you seize the opportunity it presented?

*Steps of a significant event audit*

**Step 1** Describe who was involved, what time of day, what task/activity, the context and any other relevant information.

**Step 2** Reflect on the effects of the event on yourself and others.

**Step 3** Discuss the reasons for the event or situation arising with others, review case notes or other records.

**Step 4** Decide how you or others might have behaved differently. Describe your options for how your teaching might change to minimise or eliminate the event from recurring.

**Step 5** Plan changes that are needed, how they will be implemented, who will be responsible for what and when, what further training or resources are required. Then carry out the changes.

**Step 6** Re-audit later to see whether changes to your teaching style or delivery of learning are having the desired effects.

# Examples of evidence of your competence or performance as a teacher – and how appropriate is your teaching style

The stages of the evidence cycle (see Figure 11.1) and examples that we suggest you work through in this chapter, are derived from Chambers *et al*, *Appraisal for the Apprehensive* and *Demonstrating your Competence*.[8,9]

Using the evidence cycle in Figure 11.1, here are three examples. You could replicate one or all of these three examples, or adapt them for your circumstances and needs. Or you could compose your own approach entirely. You

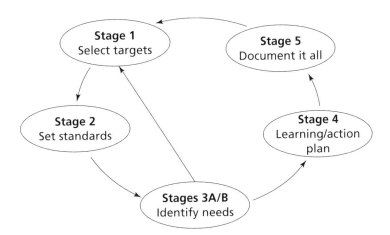

**Figure 11.1** Stages of the evidence cycle.

might consider undertaking three or four cycles of evidence per year to demonstrate your competence, or performance as a teacher and/or teaching styles you employ. If you want to know more look at the underpinning text books for more detail and guidance.[8,9]

## Example One

**Focus:** Teaching and training, combining the all-round flexible and adaptable teacher with the official curriculum teacher style.

---

**Case study 11.1 Adapting your teaching style to differing learning styles.**

Ann is apprehensive about teaching the group of junior doctors at their induction. They are expected to learn about what the Trust requires concerning human resource matters including their working hours and other employee issues. She realises that to engage the attention of the doctors, she needs to provide the information in a variety of ways to appeal to the doctors' differing learning styles.

---

This is just an example. Keep your task simple. You could choose three or four cycles of evidence to demonstrate your competence as a teacher, each year.

**Stage 1** Set your aspirations for good practice. The excellent healthcare teacher:

- uses teaching methods and a teaching style appropriate to the purpose of the teaching and the learning styles of those participating in the educational activity.

**Stage 2** Set the standards for your outcomes:
2.1 Learners gain and apply new knowledge and skills under your guidance
2.2 Flexible strategy for matching teaching style(s) to purpose of teaching and trainees' different learning styles.

Outcomes might include:
- the way learning is applied
- a learnt skill
- a protocol
- a strategy that is implemented
- meeting recommended standards

**Stage 3A** Identify your learning needs.

3A.1 Reflective diary: recording your account of teaching style you used with learners during teaching sessions and answering their queries on an everyday basis.

3A.2 Peer review of your teaching style(s): of an audio-tape or video-tape of yourself conducting a tutorial or teaching session.

**Stage 3B**. Identify your service needs.

3B.1 Review whether the learning needs of all those for whom you are responsible for teaching have been identified over last 6–12 months, and are known to you, before you embark on teaching them in a formal or informal capacity – and how you adapted your teaching style.

> Any of the needs assessment exercises in Stage 3A may also reveal service needs.

3B.2 Undertake a SWOT analysis with the line managers or educational supervisors of learners to determine whether sufficient resources are provided for the teaching methods appropriate to learning styles and the educational objectives, and the teaching style you did use and/or would prefer to use.

**Stage 4** Make and carry out a learning and action plan.

4.1 Read up on Honey and Mumford learning styles.[10]

4.2 Observe an 'expert' teacher at work with a diverse group of students. Discuss the way he/she adapted their teaching style to differing learning styles, purpose of teaching and the response from the students.

4.3 Review the audio or video tape with a peer and discuss your teaching style (see Stage 3A above).

4.4 Present your results from the SWOT analysis to the trust and/or deanery to discuss how resources for teaching can be extended and your preferred teaching style be afforded.

**Stage 5** Document your learning, competence, performance and standards of service delivery.

5.1 Repeat your observations in your reflective diary in relation to all teaching and training activities.

5.2 Repeat the SWOT analysis after changes have been made.

---

**Case study 11.1 continued**

After learning more about other people's learning styles and her preferred teaching style, Ann arranges her session with elements of the official curriculum teacher (for the first half of her teaching session) and an all-round flexible and adaptable teaching style (for the second half of her teaching session). This included a short lecture and then large group discussion about the human resources topics, small group problem solving around examples of common issues for doctors, and a handout with facts and figures.

5.3 Compare audits of a learner's practice before and after the learner has participated in a teaching session with you using your preferred teaching style.

5.4 Retain the lesson plan and notes from teaching session recording the adaptations made to trial different teaching styles and to accommodate differing styles of learning together with the feedback from the students.

## Example two

**Focus:** Teaching problem based learning on a one-off teaching style basis.

---

### Case study 11.2 Problem based learning.

Carl has been appointed as the Problem Based Learning (PBL) tutor at the local university where a medical school has just been established. His task is to teach a group of local general practitioners and primary care nurses in using the PBL approach for the medical students who will be placed in the community for a good proportion of their time. Carl is aware that the way he teaches colleagues in PBL facilitation skills is critical to their enablement of medical students' learning, and the reputation of the medical school. He is a bit apprehensive about teaching the group as he has not met them before and it will be another tutor colleague who supports the group in future as they use their problem based learning skills.

---

This is just an example. Keep your task simple. You could choose three or four cycles of evidence to demonstrate your competence as a teacher, each year.

**Stage 1** Set your aspirations for good practice. The excellent healthcare teacher who uses problem based learning:

- understands the PBL process
- employs a teaching style and skills to encourage the self directed learning crucial for the students' progress.

**Stage 2** Set the standards for your outcomes.

2.1 PBL is used appropriately to meet the learning objectives.

2.2 Use of PBL optimises the extent and depth of the students' learning.

2.3 Addressing learners' needs satisfactorily despite one-off basis of teaching relationship

Outcomes might include:
- the way learning is applied
- a learnt skill
- a protocol
- a strategy that is implemented
- meeting recommended standards

**Stage 3A** Identify your learning needs.

3A.1 Check out if you are sufficiently familiar with the process of problem based learning. You could write down the steps of the process and compare yours with the suggested stages on page 107.

3A.2 Write out three scenarios that you believe are suitable for problem based learning and ask a colleague tutor to critique your efforts and suggest revisions. Ask the tutor to comment on whether the learning objectives and problems are relevant, the problems are appropriate to curriculum and stage of learner, that there is sufficient context and depth, and the extent to which your teaching style was appropriate.

3A.3 Ask any students who you have supervised in doing PBL in the past to give you feedback in informal or formal ways about the process, the scenario, your facilitation, and the overall outcomes – to help you gain insights into the best ways to help new PBL tutors to prepare.

3A.4 Undertake a self-assessment of your preferred teaching style (see Chapter 2).

**Stage 3B** Identify your service needs.

3B.1 Compare your feedback from learners with that of other teachers involved in teaching or supporting the PBL facilitation process.

3B.2 Measure facets of students' learning and engagement; compare against the learning objectives, the organisation of learning, the

Any of the needs assessment exercises in Stage 3A may also reveal service needs.

availability of information sources and the evidence to solve the problems. Look for reasons why learners' experiences and learning outcomes might differ – in relation to a particular teaching style, the circumstances of the learner or the time spent.

**Stage 4** Make and carry out a learning and action plan.

4.1 Carrying out exercises in sections 3A and 3B will be an integral part of learning.

4.2 Read up about PBL and competencies of problem based tutors.[11,12]

4.3 Attend a workshop on the teaching of problem based learning and any support group for PBL tutors.

4.4 Attend a workshop specialising on learning about teaching styles and their potential impact in different settings with various kinds of learners.

**Stage 5** Document your learning, competence, performance and standards of service delivery.

5.1 Collect workshop notes, certificates of attendance and outstanding training needs in your continuing personal development plan.

5.2 Record the needs assessment and learning from exercises 3A.1 and 3A.2 with corrections and revisions to list of steps in PBL process and PBL scenarios.

5.3 Obtain feedback from learners engaged in teaching PBL after your tutorship.

5.4 Reflective diary records of attempts at adopting different teaching styles.

---

**Case study 11.2 continued**

Your one-off teaching style works out well. The learners are enthusiastic about the PBL approach. The excellent facilitation skills by general practitioners and primary care nurses who are well versed in the PBL process means that the medical students rate the scenarios and subsequent learning highly.

---

## Example three

**Focus:** Giving constructive feedback with a sensitive student-centred teaching style.

---

**Case study 11.3 Using feedback to help others become consciously competent.**

As a teacher of undergraduates Jed aims to help his nursing students become consciously competent in taking a child patient's clinical history by the time they leave their placement with him. When they arrive they are usually unaware of the gaps in their knowledge and skills about history taking, and the extent to which they should include both child and parent/carer in the task.

---

This is just an example. Keep your task simple. You could choose three or four cycles of evidence to demonstrate your competence as a teacher, each year.

**Stage 1** Set your aspirations for good practice. The excellent healthcare teacher is:

- able to give effective feedback to learners
- able to move unconsciously or consciously incompetent learners to conscious competence across a range of practice.

**Stage 2** Set the standards for your outcomes.
2.1 Able to identify and reduce knowledge and skill gaps and any limiting attitudes of students.
2.2 Able to adopt a student-centred sensitive teaching style effectively.

> Outcomes might include:
> - the way learning is applied
> - a learnt skill
> - a protocol
> - a strategy that is implemented
> - meeting recommended standards.

**Stage 3A** Identify your learning needs.
3A.1 Self-recognition of your own perceived weaknesses in identifying the gaps in other people's knowledge and skill.
3A.2 Compare your rating of the competence of students with that of trained colleagues – reflecting on the differences between the groups.
3A.3 Arrange an audit of a student's performance by yourself, the student and another experienced colleague in a key clinical topic or non-clinical skill (e.g. record keeping). Compare your audit results and their interpretation considering knowledge, skills and attitude.

**Stage 3B** Identify your service needs.
3B.1 Consider adverse comments or feedback made about a student by a child patient, their parents/carers or staff and your own role and responsibility as a teacher and style of teaching.
3B.2 Arrange multisource feedback from colleagues about your teaching style and ability to motivate others in relation to learning and performance improvement.

> Any of the needs assessment exercises in Stage 3A may also reveal service needs.

**Stage 4** Make and carry out a learning and action plan.
4.1 Read up about the Johari window model.[13] Discuss and reflect on the contents with colleagues.
4.2 Go on a course in motivational skills.
4.3 Undertake a postgraduate award in medical education.
4.4 Review problem issues relating to your competence or teaching style using case studies with teacher/trainer colleague.

**Stage 5** Document your learning, competence, performance and standards of service delivery.
5.1 Document the review of problem issues relating to your competence or teaching style using case studies with teacher/trainer colleague.

5.2 Record changes in knowledge, skills and behaviour of students.

5.3 Repeat one or more learning or service needs exercises described in sections 3A or 3B above and make comparison with the baseline.

---

**Case study 11.3 continued**

By the time the students leave their placement they have become consciously competent at history taking in relation to a general paediatrics clinical setting. They have their checklists of questions to progress through and are competent at probing further if the patient or parent/carer describes important symptoms. You have evidence from the multisource feedback and your own reflections confirm that you are indeed an effective teacher when you adopt a sensitive student-centred teaching style.

---

# References

1 Donaldson L. *Good doctors, safer patients.* A consultation. London: DH; 2006.

2 Department of Health. *The regulation of the non-medical healthcare professions.* A consultation. London: DH; 2006.

3 Nursing and Midwifery Council. *Code of Professional Conduct.* London: Nursing and Midwifery Council; 2002.

4 General Medical Council. *Good Medical Practice.* London: General Medical Council; 2006.

5 Royal College of General Practitioners. *Portfolio-based Learning in General Practice.* Occasional Paper 63. London: RCGP; 1993.

6 Eraut M, du Boulay B. Developing the attributes of medical professional judgement and competence. Sussex: University of Sussex; 2000. Reproduced at www.cogs.susx.ac.uk/users/bend/doh

7 Fraser SW, Greenhalgh T. Coping with complexity: educating for capability. *BMJ.* 2001; **323**: 799–803.

8 Chambers R, Wakley G, Field S, *et al. Appraisal for the Apprehensive.* Oxford: Radcliffe Medical Press; 2002.

9 Chambers R, Mohanna K, Wakley G, *et al. Demonstrating your competence 1: healthcare teaching.* Oxford: Radcliffe Medical Press; 2004.

10 Honey P, Mumford A. *Using Your Learning Styles.* Maidenhead: Peter Honey Publications; 1986.

11 Barrow HS. A taxonomy of problem-based learning methods. *Med Educ.* 1986; **20**: 481–6.

12 Hughes L, Lucas J. An evaluation of problem based learning in the multiprofessional education curriculum for the health professions. *J Interprof Care.* 1997; **11**: 77–88.

13 Luft J. *Group processes: an introduction to group dynamics.* Palo Alto, Calif: National Press Books; 1970.

# Appendix: Background to the research to derive the Staffordshire Evaluation of Teaching Styles

## Introduction

We were looking to find styles that individual teachers were comfortable using in their teaching. Teaching style is likely to be influenced by several factors, including comfort with using the style, capacity to use the style, and organisational expectations and limitations within the system that the teacher is working in.

## Aim

*Preferred teaching styles* were our interest here. Was it possible to derive a valid self-assessment tool that was simple to administer and that could reliably discriminate between teachers with different preferences?

## Method

We undertook an electronic literature search of PubMed, EMBASE, CINAHL and ERIC databases and further hand searches in 2004. Search terms included: doctor, peer review, competence, capability, competency, education, teaching, training, teaching styles. We confined the literature to that specifically relating to healthcare teachers. From those papers identified as relevant to our study's aims we extracted all descriptions of any aspects of teaching styles or delivery of healthcare teaching. We identified key themes and constructed a series of paired questions hoping to define differences between these aspects. We constructed an initial four page questionnaire, containing 96 paired key statements about teaching styles, using a 1–5 Likert scale format for each statement.

A period of consultation with fellow healthcare teachers followed and this refined the questions until we could be sure that all themes that could be considered to be part of a definition of teaching styles were included. This took the form of a modified Delphi technique with 20 individual clinicians working in medical education. We asked for opinions on the initial questionnaire, including the design, the content, and any obvious gaps or duplications. Some respondents wanted to know their own teaching styles at this stage, giving us encouragement that such a tool was needed.

The full questionnaire was piloted on 10 medical and dental educators to test the process, to test the questionnaire and to test the approach to the statistical analysis. With some modification in the light of this, we mailed the questionnaire to a total of 132 medical and dental educators using the West Midlands Deanery database of educators. Respondents were asked to rate a series of 96 statements and to indicate for each one 'how relevant the statement was in describing them as a teacher of an undergraduate or postgraduate student, or health professional or manager undertaking continuing professional development'.

We also asked each contributor about their educational post, what discipline they worked in, their main job or post, medical school of qualification, year of qualification and gender.

## Results

A total of 88 individuals out of 132 from a variety of backgrounds within medical and dental education in the West Midlands answered this questionnaire, a 67% response rate.

There were 65 male and 23 female responders. Of these, there were 53 general practitioners, 12 dentists, 22 consultants and 1 nurse practitioner. Most had been qualified over 25 years, as can be seen from Figure A.1.

The results were analysed using SPSS for basic frequencies (numbers in each category), for reliability analysis and using principal component factor analysis.

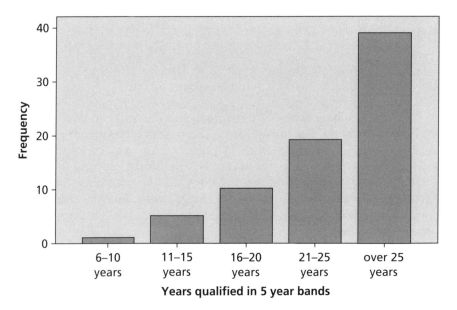

**Figure A.1** Age distribution of medical and dental educator respondents.

Reliability for our data was very good with an overall Cronbach's alpha of 0.901. There were no questions which stood out as being of poor reliability using the 'alpha if item deleted' function in the calculations of reliability. (Cronbach's alpha is a measure of how internally consistent the data is as a whole. The value of Cronbach's alpha may vary from zero (no consistency at all) through to one (perfect internal consistency). In practice, a value of 0.7 or above is normally taken as being sufficiently reliable for research purposes, and a value of 0.8 as being sufficiently reliable for pass/fail examination purposes.)

In order to group the data from these 96 questions into different teaching styles with descriptive statements attached to each one, 'factor analysis' was used. (Factor analysis is a statistical technique which groups together questions which are answered in a similar way by responders, by first constructing a correlation matrix of all questions, and then extracting factors from the correlation matrix based on the correlation coefficients of the question scores. The factors are rotated in order to maximise the relationship between the results of the questions and some of the factors. Individual questions may load onto the different factors, some more strongly than others.)

We used an exploratory factor analysis (to explore relationships within the Likert data) using principal component factor analysis, with varimax rotation and with Kaiser normalisation. The number of factors (and therefore for us how many teaching styles) to be accepted is a matter of debate and of judgement.[1] There are two main methods of doing this. On the one hand there is the Kaiser criterion,[2] accepting all factors with an Eigen value of above 1.0, which would have given 26 different factors (and 26 different teaching styles – far too many to be really useful for our purposes.) Instead, we used the

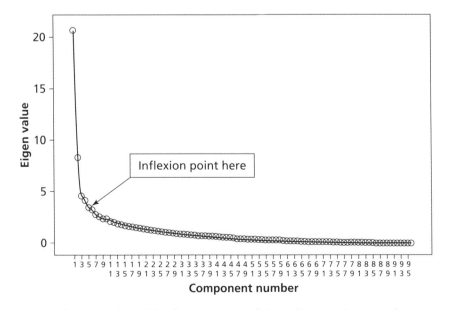

**Figure A.2** The scree plot of the factors extracted from the questionnaire data.

second method described by Cattell, using a scree plot and determining the number of factors by the inflexion point in the scree plot curve, and accepting all factors above that point.[3] This inflexion point was achieved with six factors, and setting SPSS to accept these six factors produced a convergence within 12 iterations. Eigen values for all these factors were above 3.0, when the curve levelled out into 'scree'. Figure A2 shows the scree plot of factors from our data.

What is also shown in the results of the factor analysis is how the questions load onto each of the six factors, and which questions load most strongly onto each factor, so we can then say something about what each factor is about. In fact we took the strongest loaded four questions for each factor to provide a descriptor for each factor.

We labelled the six factors as follows:

1 the all-round flexible and adaptable teacher
2 the student-centred, sensitive teacher
3 the official curriculum teacher
4 the straight facts no nonsense teacher
5 the big conference teacher
6 the one-off teacher.

# Linking the six factors with different characteristics of our respondents

Once we had the six factors decided and defined, it was then possible to test statistically which other variables in our respondents (educational post, clinical discipline the individual was working in, the main job or post, medical school of qualification, year of qualification and gender) were loaded onto each of the six factors. The statistical tests used were ANOVA and Kruskall Wallis tests, again using SPSS.

In terms of clinical discipline, the clinical job did indeed make a difference. The student-centred, sensitive teacher was strongest for general practitioners, with a p value of 0.049. The official curriculum teacher was strongest for dentists, with a p value of 0.014. The big conference teacher was strongest for medical consultants, with a p value of 0.007, highly significant.

In terms of years qualified in five year bands, there were no differences in any of the six styles. In terms of place of basic medical qualification there were no differences.

By gender, the only one of the six factors which showed a significant difference was in the big conference teacher factor, which was strongest for males, with a p value of 0.025.

# Constructing the self evaluation questionnaire

To create a more user friendly tool, we developed a 24 item self evaluation questionnaire using the four strongest loaded Likert statements for each of the six styles. A random numbers table was used to determine the position of each of the statements in the self evaluation questionnaire to avoid putting all four items of one style together.

The Staffordshire Hexagon presentation of results offers a representation of a respondent's relative strength in each teaching style based on their scores. It will then be easily seen which are the preferred styles with the highest scores, and which are the least preferred styles with the lowest scores.

So far we have begun to discern several patterns of styles. This is part of further research work to see if there are major differences between different groups of teachers in different clinical disciplines and different professions. This is ongoing, and at present we have no definite answers.

# References

1   Field A. *Discovering statistics using SPSS for Windows*. London: Sage Publications Limited; 2000.

2   Kaiser HF. The application of electronic computers to factor analysis. *Educ Psychol Meas*. 1960; **20**: 141–51.

3   Cattell RB. The scree test for a number of factors. *Multivar Behav Res*. 1966; **1**, 245–76.

# Index